Face Yoga Book

A Comprehensive Guide to Facial Exercises and Techniques.

Enhancing Your Face Yoga Practice with Face Oils.

Maia Sobinina

Girls are Gorgeous

Keep informed about our newest and
updated developments by scanning this
QR code.

DEDICATION

To my loved ones - family, friends, and mankind - this book is dedicated to you. You are the source of my inspiration and motivation, and your love and support has made this project possible. Thank you for believing in me and for being a constant source of encouragement. May this book bring joy and positive change to your lives and to the lives of all those who read it.

Acknowledgments:

Writing this book would not have been possible without the support and encouragement of many individuals. I would like to express my heartfelt gratitude to the following people for their contributions:

- *My family, for their unwavering love and support throughout this journey. Your encouragement and belief in me have been invaluable.*

My friends, for their constant encouragement and for being a sounding board for my ideas.

- *My editor, for their insightful feedback and for helping me to refine my thoughts and ideas.*
- *The experts and professionals in the field of skincare and wellness, for sharing their knowledge and expertise.*
- *All those who have supported and inspired me along the way, thank you for your contributions to this project.*

Lastly, I would like to thank my readers for choosing this book and for supporting my work. It is my hope that this book will bring joy and positive change to your lives.

Table of Contents

Chapter 1: Introducing the concept of Face Yoga and how it can benefit the skin. Discussing the benefits of using face oils in conjunction with Face Yoga.

In recent years, there has been a growing trend in the beauty industry that involves using exercises and techniques to improve the health and appearance of the skin. One such trend is Face Yoga, which involves a series of exercises that target the muscles in the face, neck, and head. The goal of Face Yoga is to tone and tighten the skin to create a more youthful appearance. However, Face Yoga can be even more effective when paired with the use of face oils. In this chapter, we'll introduce the concept of Face Yoga and explore how it can benefit the skin when used in conjunction with face oils.

The concept of Face Yoga is based on the idea that, like any other muscles in the body, the facial muscles can be toned and strengthened through exercise. By performing regular facial exercises, individuals can help to reduce the signs of aging, such as wrinkles and sagging, and promote a more youthful and vibrant appearance.

While the practice of Face Yoga is relatively new, the principles behind it are rooted in ancient practices such as yoga and Ayurveda. In traditional yoga, certain postures and breathing exercises are believed to promote health and vitality throughout the body, including the face. Ayurveda, an ancient Indian system of medicine, also emphasizes the importance of maintaining balance and harmony in the body and mind for optimal health, which includes the health of the face.

In Face Yoga, exercises are designed to target specific areas of the face, such as the forehead, eyes, cheeks, and chin, to improve muscle tone and circulation. Techniques such as massage, acupressure, and relaxation exercises may also be incorporated to promote relaxation and reduce tension and stress in the face and scalp.

Benefits of Face Yoga include improved skin tone, reduction of wrinkles and fine lines, increased circulation, and overall facial rejuvenation. Additionally, Face Yoga may also help to promote relaxation, reduce stress, and improve overall well-being.

What is Face Yoga?

Face Yoga is a natural and non-invasive alternative to more invasive cosmetic procedures, such as Botox and facelifts, which can be costly and carry risks and side effects. With regular practice, Face Yoga can help individuals to achieve a more youthful and radiant appearance, without the need for expensive treatments or surgery.

The exercises are designed to increase blood flow to the muscles, which can help to nourish them and promote healthy cell growth. Additionally, the movements involved in Face Yoga can help to strengthen and tone the muscles, which can give the skin a firmer, more lifted appearance.

The Benefits of Using Face Oils

Face oils are a popular skincare product that can be used to moisturize and nourish the skin. They are made from a combination of natural oils and can help to improve the overall health and appearance of the skin. Here are some of the benefits of using face oils in conjunction with Face Yoga:

1. **Improved hydration:** Face oils can help to lock in moisture and keep the skin hydrated, which is important for maintaining a youthful appearance.

2. **Increased nourishment:** Face oils contain a variety of vitamins and nutrients that can help to nourish the skin and promote healthy cell growth.

3. **Reduced inflammation:** Many face oils contain anti-inflammatory ingredients that can help to reduce redness and inflammation in the skin.

4. **Enhanced absorption:** When used in conjunction with Face Yoga, face oils can help to enhance the absorption of nutrients into the skin.

5. **Improved overall skin health:** By moisturizing and nourishing the skin, face oils can help to improve the overall health and appearance of the skin.

Face Yoga and face oils can work together to provide a natural and holistic approach to facial health and rejuvenation. Face oils are plant-based oils that are rich in nutrients, antioxidants, and fatty acids, which can help to nourish and hydrate the skin. When combined with Face Yoga exercises, face oils can help to improve skin tone, reduce the signs of aging, and promote overall facial health.

The use of face oils in Face Yoga can help to enhance the benefits of the exercises. When applied to the skin before or after performing Face Yoga exercises, face oils can help to provide a barrier that locks in moisture and nutrients, while also protecting the skin from environmental stressors. Additionally, the massaging and acupressure techniques used in Face Yoga can help to stimulate blood flow and promote the absorption of the oils into the skin.

There are a variety of face oils available on the market, each with its unique properties and benefits. Some popular face oils include jojoba oil, rosehip oil, and argan oil. When selecting a face oil for use in Face Yoga, it is important to choose one that is appropriate for your skin type and concerns.

When incorporating face oils into your Face Yoga routine, it is important to apply them correctly. Begin by cleansing your face and applying any serums or toners before applying the face oil. Use a few drops of the oil and gently massage it into the skin using upward and outward motions. Allow the oil to absorb before beginning your Face Yoga exercises.

In conclusion, the use of face oils in conjunction with Face Yoga can provide a natural and effective approach to facial health and rejuvenation. By nourishing and hydrating the skin with face oils and stimulating blood flow through Face Yoga exercises, individuals can achieve a more youthful and radiant appearance. When selecting face oils for use in Face Yoga, be sure to choose one that is appropriate for your skin type and needs, and always apply them correctly for maximum benefits.

Chapter 2. The Benefits of Face Oils: Discussing the benefits of using face oils on the skin, including how they can help to moisturize, nourish, and protect the skin.

Face oils have become increasingly popular in the world of skincare, providing a natural and effective way to nourish, hydrate, and protect the skin. Unlike traditional moisturizers, which are often water-based, face oils are made from plant-based oils that are rich in nutrients, antioxidants, and fatty acids that can help to improve the health and appearance of the skin.

The use of face oils in skincare is not a new concept. In fact, many ancient cultures used oils to promote skin health and beauty. In recent years, face oils have regained popularity as consumers seek out more natural and holistic approaches to skincare.

Face oils:

Moisturize the Skin

One of the primary benefits of face oils is their ability to moisturize the skin. Face oils are rich in fatty acids, which can help to create a protective barrier on the skin's surface, preventing moisture loss and keeping the skin hydrated. This can be particularly beneficial for those with dry or dehydrated skin, as face oils can help to improve the skin's texture and appearance.

Nourish the Skin

In addition to moisturizing the skin, face oils can also provide essential nutrients that can help to nourish and repair the skin. Many face oils contain vitamins, such as vitamin E and C, that can help to protect the skin from environmental stressors, promote collagen production, and reduce the appearance of fine lines and wrinkles.

Face oils are rich in nutrients, antioxidants, and fatty acids, which help to nourish and hydrate the skin. The fatty acids in face oils help to strengthen the skin barrier, reducing moisture loss and preventing dehydration. Additionally, the antioxidants in face oils can help to protect the skin from environmental stressors, such as pollution and UV rays, which can lead to premature aging.

Protect the Skin

Face oils can also provide a protective layer on the skin, which can help to shield it from environmental damage. Many face oils contain antioxidants that can help to neutralize free radicals, which are unstable molecules that can damage the skin and cause premature aging.

Help to Balance Oil Production

Contrary to popular belief, using face oils can actually help to balance oil production in the skin. When the skin is dehydrated, it can produce more oil in an attempt to compensate for the lack of moisture. By moisturizing the skin with face oils, it can help to regulate the skin's oil production and prevent excess oiliness.

Suitable for All Skin Types

Face oils are versatile and can be used by individuals with all skin types. Those with oily skin may benefit from lightweight, non-comedogenic oils such as jojoba or rosehip oil, while those with dry skin may prefer richer oils such as argan or marula oil. Additionally, face oils can be used on sensitive skin as they are generally non-irritating and hypoallergenic.

Improve Skin Texture and Tone

Face oils can help to improve the texture and tone of the skin. They can help to reduce the appearance of fine lines and wrinkles, improve skin elasticity, and promote a more radiant and youthful complexion.

Balance the Skin

Some face oils, such as jojoba oil, have a structure similar to the natural oils produced by the skin. By applying these oils to the skin, they can help to balance the skin's natural oil production and reduce the appearance of oily skin.

Sooth Irritated Skin

Face oils can help to soothe and calm irritated or inflamed skin. Oils like chamomile and lavender have anti-inflammatory properties that can help to reduce redness and inflammation.

Versatile

Face oils are versatile and can be used in a variety of ways. They can be used alone or in combination with other skincare products, such as moisturizers and serums, to enhance their benefits. Additionally, many face oils can be used on other areas of the body, such as the hair and nails, to promote overall health and beauty.

Affordable

Face oils are often more affordable than traditional skincare products, making them a great option for those on a budget.

Face oils come in a variety of formulations, each with its unique properties and benefits. Some popular face oils include jojoba oil, rosehip oil, and argan oil. When selecting a face oil, it is important to consider your skin type and concerns, as well as the specific properties and benefits of the oil.

One of the benefits of using face oils is their ability to penetrate deeply into the skin and provide long-lasting hydration. The fatty acids in face oils help to strengthen the skin barrier, reducing moisture loss and preventing dehydration. Additionally, the antioxidants in face oils can help to protect the skin from environmental stressors, such as pollution and UV rays, which can lead to premature aging.

Another benefit of face oils is their versatility. They can be used alone or in combination with other skincare products, such as moisturizers and serums, to enhance their benefits. Additionally, many face oils can be used on other areas of the body, such as the hair and nails, to promote overall health and beauty.

To use face oils, simply apply a few drops to your fingertips and gently massage into the skin using upward and outward motions. Face oils can be used in the morning or evening, depending on your preference and skincare routine.

In conclusion, face oils offer a natural and effective way to nourish and protect the skin. With their rich nutrients and antioxidants, face oils can help to improve skin hydration, reduce the signs of aging, and promote a more radiant and youthful complexion. When selecting a face oil, consider your skin type and concerns, and always apply the oil correctly for maximum benefits.

Chapter 3. The Best Face Oils for Face Yoga: The best types of face oils to use for Face Yoga, including their unique properties and benefits.

Face Yoga is a natural and effective way to improve the health and appearance of the skin. When paired with the right face oil, the benefits of Face Yoga can be even greater. Face oils are rich in vitamins, antioxidants, and essential fatty acids that can help to moisturize, nourish, and protect the skin. However, not all face oils are created equal, and some may be more beneficial for Face Yoga than others. In this chapter, we'll outline the best types of face oils to use for Face Yoga, including their unique properties and benefits.

1. Jojoba Oil

Jojoba oil is a lightweight, non-comedogenic oil that is easily absorbed by the skin. It is rich in vitamin E and B-complex vitamins, which can help to nourish and protect the skin. Jojoba oil also has anti-inflammatory properties, which can help to reduce redness and inflammation in the skin. For those with oily or acne-prone skin, jojoba oil is an excellent choice as it can help to regulate oil production and prevent clogged pores.

2. Rosehip Oil

Rosehip oil is a rich source of vitamin C, which can help to brighten the skin and improve collagen production. It is also high in essential fatty acids, which can help to hydrate and nourish the skin. Rosehip oil has been shown to have anti-aging properties, as it can help to reduce the appearance of fine lines and wrinkles. For those with dry or mature skin, rosehip oil is an excellent choice as it can help to improve skin elasticity and promote a more youthful appearance.

3. Argan Oil

Argan oil is a rich source of vitamin E and essential fatty acids, which can help to moisturize and nourish the skin. It also contains antioxidants, which can help to protect the skin from environmental stressors. Argan oil has been shown to have anti-inflammatory properties, making it an excellent choice for those with sensitive or irritated skin. For those with combination skin, argan oil is an excellent choice as it can help to balance oil production and improve overall skin health.

4. Marula Oil

Marula oil is rich in antioxidants and essential fatty acids, which can help to nourish and protect the skin. It is also high in vitamin C, which can help to brighten the skin and improve collagen production. Marula oil has been shown to have anti-inflammatory properties, making it an excellent choice for those with sensitive or irritated skin. For those with dry or mature skin, marula oil is an excellent choice as it can help to improve skin elasticity and promote a more youthful appearance.

5. Oil Blends

The best face oils are often a combination of several oils, each with their own unique benefits. This allows for a synergistic effect, where the combined ingredients work together to provide maximum benefits for the skin.

For example, a face oil that contains a combination of jojoba oil, rosehip oil, and argan oil, is a popular and effective blend. Jojoba oil is a light and non-greasy oil that closely mimics the skin's natural sebum, making it highly compatible with the skin. Rosehip oil is rich in antioxidants and fatty acids, making it ideal for nourishing and restoring the skin. Argan oil is high in vitamin E and essential fatty acids, making it excellent for improving skin texture and reducing the appearance of fine lines and wrinkles.

Another popular combination is lavender oil and chamomile oil, which are both known for their calming and soothing properties. Lavender oil is also antimicrobial, making it ideal for treating acne-prone skin. Chamomile oil is also known for its anti-inflammatory properties, making it an excellent choice for those with sensitive skin.

A face oil that contains a combination of evening primrose oil and calendula oil is another popular blend. Evening primrose oil is high in essential fatty acids, making it ideal for nourishing and hydrating the skin. Calendula oil is known for its healing properties and is particularly effective for soothing and calming irritated skin.

The best face oils are often a combination of several oils, each with their own unique benefits.

When selecting a face oil to use with Face Yoga, it is important to consider your skin type and concerns. For example, if you have oily or acne-prone skin, you may want to choose a lightweight oil like jojoba oil. If you are concerned about reducing the signs of aging, a face oil like rosehip oil or marula oil may be a good choice.

To use a face oil with Face Yoga, simply apply a few drops of the oil to your fingertips and massage into the skin using upward and outward motions. The massaging and acupressure techniques used in Face Yoga can help to stimulate blood flow and promote the absorption of the oil into the skin.

In conclusion, face oils offer a natural and effective way to nourish, hydrate, and protect the skin. Whether you choose jojoba oil, rosehip oil, argan oil, marula oil, or coconut oil, the right face oil can help to improve skin texture and tone, balance the skin, soothe irritated skin, and provide overall facial health. When selecting a face oil, consider your skin type and concerns, and always apply the oil correctly for maximum benefits.

Chapter 4. The Science of Face Yoga: Exploring the science behind Face Yoga, including how it can help to improve circulation, tone facial muscles, and reduce the signs of aging.

As we age, the skin on our face naturally loses its elasticity and firmness, leading to wrinkles, fine lines, and other signs of aging. However, there is a growing trend in the beauty industry that claims to help combat these signs: Face Yoga. Face Yoga involves a series of exercises that target the muscles in the face, neck, and head, with the goal of toning and tightening the skin to create a more youthful appearance. But does the science support the claims of Face Yoga? In this chapter, we'll explore the science behind Face Yoga and how it can help to improve circulation, tone facial muscles, and reduce the signs of aging.

The Science Behind Face Yoga

To understand how Face Yoga works, it's helpful to first understand the anatomy of the face. The face contains over 43 different muscles, each with its own function, such as helping us to smile, frown, or raise our eyebrows. These muscles are connected to the skin and underlying tissue, which gives our face its shape and structure.

Just like any other muscle in our body, the muscles in our face can become weak and lose tone over time. This is due to a combination of factors, including natural aging, stress, and lack of exercise. When these muscles weaken, the skin on top of them becomes more prone to wrinkles, sagging, and other signs of aging.

Face Yoga aims to combat these effects by targeting the muscles in the face with specific exercises. These exercises are designed to increase blood flow to the muscles, which can help to nourish them and promote healthy cell growth. Additionally, the movements involved in Face Yoga can help to strengthen and tone the muscles, which can give the skin a firmer, more lifted appearance.

Incorporating facial exercises into your skincare routine can offer numerous advantages, including strengthened muscles, increased blood flow, and reduced stress. Practicing Face Yoga regularly can help maintain a youthful and glowing complexion. Here are the potential benefits:

1. **Increased circulation:** When we exercise any muscle in our body, it increases blood flow to that area. The same is true for the muscles in our face. By practicing Face Yoga regularly, we can increase blood flow to these muscles, which can help to nourish them and promote healthy cell growth.

2. **Toned facial muscles:** The movements involved in Face Yoga can help to strengthen and tone the muscles in the face, which can give the skin a firmer, more lifted appearance. This can help to reduce the appearance of sagging skin and wrinkles.

3. **Reduced stress and tension:** Many of the exercises in Face Yoga involve deep breathing and relaxation techniques, which can help to reduce stress and tension in the face and neck. This can help to prevent the formation of wrinkles and other signs of aging caused by stress.

4. **Improved lymphatic drainage:** The lymphatic system is responsible for removing waste and toxins from the body.

By practicing Face Yoga, we can help to stimulate lymphatic drainage in the face, which can help to reduce puffiness and inflammation.

5. **Natural alternative to invasive procedures:** While there are many cosmetic procedures available to help reduce the signs of aging, these can be expensive and come with potential risks and side effects. Face Yoga offers a natural, non-invasive alternative that can help to improve the health and appearance of the skin.

Conclusion

By incorporating Face Yoga into your skincare routine, you may be able to achieve a more youthful, radiant complexion without the need for invasive procedures or expensive creams. As with any exercise program, it's important to consult with a healthcare professional.

Chapter 5. The Fundamentals of Face Yoga: The basic techniques and exercises of Face Yoga, including facial massage, facial exercises, and acupressure.

If you're interested in trying Face Yoga to improve the health and appearance of your skin, it's important to start with the fundamentals. These basic techniques and exercises form the foundation of any Face Yoga practice, and can help to improve circulation, tone facial muscles, and reduce the signs of aging. In this chapter, we'll explore the fundamentals of Face Yoga, including facial massage, facial exercises, and acupressure.

Facial Massage

Facial massage is a key component of any Face Yoga practice. Massaging the muscles in your face can help to increase blood flow, reduce tension, and promote relaxation. Here are some basic facial massage techniques to try:

1. **The forehead:** Use your fingertips to massage your forehead in small circular motions. Start at the center of your forehead and work your way outwards.

2. **The cheeks:** Use the pads of your fingers to massage your cheeks in upward and outward motions. Start at the center of your cheeks and work your way outwards.

3. **The chin and jawline:** Use your fingertips to massage your chin and jawline in small circular motions. Start at the center of your chin and work your way outwards towards your ears.

4. **The temples:** Use your fingertips to massage your temples in small circular motions. This can help to reduce tension and headaches.

Facial Exercises

Facial exercises are another important component of Face Yoga. These exercises are designed to strengthen and tone the muscles in your face, which can help to reduce the appearance of wrinkles and sagging skin. Here are some basic facial exercises to try:

1. **The V:** Make a V shape with your fingers and place them on the corners of your mouth. Smile as wide as you can, then relax. Repeat 10 times.

2. **The fish face:** Suck in your cheeks and pucker your lips to create a fish face. Hold for 5 seconds, then relax. Repeat 10 times.

3. **The neck lift: Tilt** your head back and look up at the ceiling. Press your tongue to the roof of your mouth and hold for 5 seconds. Relax and repeat 10 times.

4. **The eyebrow lift:** Place your index fingers just above your eyebrows. Use your fingers to lift your eyebrows up as high as you can. Hold for 5 seconds, then relax. Repeat 10 times.

Acupressure

Acupressure is a technique that involves applying pressure to specific points on the body to promote healing and relaxation. In Face Yoga, acupressure is used to stimulate the flow of energy, or chi, in the face and improve overall skin health. Here are some acupressure points to try:

1. **The third eye:** Place your index and middle fingers between your eyebrows, where your third eye would be. Apply gentle pressure for 30 seconds.

2. **The temples:** Use your index and middle fingers to massage your temples in small circular motions. This can help to reduce tension and headaches.

3. **The jawline:** Use your index and middle fingers to apply gentle pressure to the points just below your earlobes. This can help to reduce tension in the jawline.

4. **The cheekbones:** Use your index and middle fingers to apply gentle pressure to the points just below your cheekbones. This can help to promote circulation and improve skin tone.

Conclusion

Facial massage, facial exercises, and acupressure are the fundamental techniques of Face Yoga. By incorporating these techniques into your skincare routine, you can help to improve circulation, tone facial muscles, and reduce the signs of aging. As with any exercise program, it's important to start slowly and listen to your body. With consistent practice, you may start to notice improvements in the health and appearance of your skin.

Chapter 6. Targeted Face Yoga Routines: Providing targeted Face Yoga routines for different skin concerns, such as wrinkles, sagging skin, and dark circles.

Face Yoga is a natural and effective way to improve the health and appearance of your skin. By incorporating targeted Face Yoga routines into your skincare routine, you can address specific skin concerns, such as wrinkles, sagging skin, and dark circles. In this chapter, we'll provide targeted Face Yoga routines for different skin concerns.

For Wrinkles:

1. **Forehead massage:** Use your fingertips to massage your forehead in small circular motions, starting at the center and working your way outwards. This can help to reduce tension and wrinkles in the forehead.

2. **The V:** Make a V shape with your fingers and place them on the corners of your mouth. Smile as wide as you can, then relax. Repeat 10 times. This exercise can help to reduce wrinkles around the mouth and chin.

3. **The forehead press:** Place your fingertips on your forehead and apply gentle pressure. Slowly move your fingertips down towards your eyebrows, pressing gently. This can help to reduce wrinkles in the forehead.

4. **The eye squeeze:** Close your eyes tightly, then release. Repeat 10 times. This exercise can help to reduce wrinkles around the eyes.

For Sagging Skin:

1. **The neck lift:** Tilt your head back and look up at the ceiling. Press your tongue to the roof of your mouth and hold for 5 seconds. Relax and repeat 10 times. This exercise can help to tone the muscles in the neck and prevent sagging skin.

2. **The cheek lift:** Place your index fingers just below your cheekbones. Use your fingers to lift your cheeks up as high as you can. Hold for 5 seconds, then relax. Repeat 10 times. This exercise can help to lift and tone the cheeks.

3. **The jawline lift:** Place your index fingers on the points just below your earlobes. Use your fingers to gently pull your skin upwards, towards your ears. Hold for 5 seconds, then relax. Repeat 10 times. This exercise can help to tone the muscles in the jawline and prevent sagging skin.

For Dark Circles:

1. **The eye massage:** Use your fingertips to massage the skin around your eyes in small circular motions. This can help to improve circulation and reduce puffiness and dark circles.

2. **The eyebrow lift:** Place your index fingers just above your eyebrows. Use your fingers to lift your eyebrows up as high as you can. Hold for 5 seconds, then relax. Repeat 10 times. This exercise can help to reduce the appearance of dark circles and puffiness around the eyes.

3. **The third eye press:** Place your index and middle fingers between your eyebrows, where your third eye would be. Apply gentle pressure for 30 seconds. This can help to improve circulation and reduce the appearance of dark circles.

Conclusion

Incorporating targeted Face Yoga routines into your skincare routine can help to address specific skin concerns, such as wrinkles, sagging skin, and dark circles. By practicing these exercises regularly, you can improve the health and appearance of your skin in a natural and non-invasive way. Remember, consistency is key when it comes to Face Yoga, so make sure to incorporate these exercises into your daily routine for best results.

Chapter 7. Incorporating Face Yoga and Face Oils into Your Daily Routine: Offering tips on how to incorporate Face Yoga and face oils into your daily skincare routine for maximum benefits.

Incorporating Face Yoga and face oils into your daily skincare routine can help to improve the health and appearance of your skin in a natural and effective way. However, it can be difficult to know where to start and how to fit these practices into your daily routine. In this chapter, we'll offer tips on how to incorporate Face Yoga and face oils into your daily routine for maximum benefits.

1. Start with a Clean Slate

Before you begin your Face Yoga routine, it's important to start with a clean slate. Make sure to cleanse your skin thoroughly to remove any makeup, dirt, or oil that may be on the surface of your skin. This will ensure that your Face Yoga and face oil practices are as effective as possible.

2. Use Face Oils in Conjunction with Face Yoga

Face oils can be used in conjunction with Face Yoga to enhance the benefits of both practices. Apply a few drops of your favorite face oil to your fingertips and massage it into your skin using gentle upward strokes. This will help to nourish and protect your skin while also providing a slip for your fingers during Face Yoga exercises.

3. Incorporate Face Yoga into Your Morning Routine

Incorporating Face Yoga into your morning routine is a great way to start the day off on the right foot. Set aside a few minutes each morning to practice facial massage, facial exercises, and acupressure. Not only will this help to improve the health and appearance of your skin, but it can also help to promote relaxation and reduce stress.

4. Practice Face Yoga in the Evening

In addition to incorporating Face Yoga into your morning routine, practicing Face Yoga in the evening can also be beneficial. Set aside a few minutes each evening to practice facial massage, facial exercises, and acupressure. This can help to relax your facial muscles and promote better sleep.

5. Make it a Habit

Consistency is key when it comes to Face Yoga and face oils. Make it a habit to practice these techniques daily for best results. Whether you choose to incorporate them into your morning or evening routine, or both, make sure to stick to your routine for at least a few weeks to see the results.

Conclusion

Incorporating Face Yoga and face oils into your daily skincare routine can help to improve the health and appearance of your skin in a natural and effective way. By starting with a clean slate, using face oils in conjunction with Face Yoga, incorporating these practices into your morning and evening routines, and making it a habit, you can enjoy the many benefits of these practices for years to come. Remember, consistency is key, so make sure to stick to your routine for best results.

Chapter 8. The Mind-Body Connection: Exploring the connection between the mind and body, and how Face Yoga and face oils can help to promote relaxation and reduce stress.

The mind and body are intimately connected, and the health of one can greatly impact the other. Stress and anxiety, for example, can manifest in physical symptoms such as muscle tension, headaches, and skin issues. On the other hand, practices such as Face Yoga and the use of face oils can help to promote relaxation and reduce stress, benefiting both the mind and body. In this chapter, we'll explore the mind-body connection and how Face Yoga and face oils can help to promote relaxation and reduce stress.

The Mind-Body Connection

The mind-body connection refers to the relationship between our thoughts, emotions, and physical health. The way we think and feel can impact our physical health, and vice versa. For example, chronic stress can lead to physical symptoms such as headaches, muscle tension, and skin issues. On the other hand, practices such as meditation, yoga, and deep breathing can help to reduce stress and promote relaxation, benefiting both the mind and body.

Face Yoga and Relaxation

Face Yoga is a practice that involves a series of facial exercises, massage techniques, and acupressure to promote the health and appearance of the skin. In addition to its physical benefits, Face Yoga can also help to promote relaxation and reduce stress. By focusing on the movements of the facial muscles and the sensations in the body, Face Yoga can help to bring your attention to the present moment and promote a sense of calm.

Facial Massage and Stress Reduction

Facial massage is a key component of Face Yoga, and it can also be used on its own to promote relaxation and reduce stress. By using gentle pressure and circular motions to massage the muscles in the face and neck, facial massage can help to relieve tension and promote a sense of relaxation. It can also help to improve circulation and promote lymphatic drainage, which can reduce puffiness and promote a more youthful appearance.

Face Oils and Aromatherapy

In addition to their nourishing and protective properties for the skin, face oils can also be used for aromatherapy to promote relaxation and reduce stress. Many face oils, such as lavender and chamomile, have calming properties and can help to promote relaxation when applied to the skin. Simply apply a few drops of your favorite face oil to your fingertips, inhale deeply, and take a moment to focus on your breath.

Conclusion

The mind and body are intimately connected, and practices such as Face Yoga and the use of face oils can help to promote relaxation and reduce stress. By bringing your attention to the present moment, focusing on the movements of the facial muscles, and using gentle pressure and circular motions to massage the muscles in the face and neck, you can promote a sense of calm and relaxation. Incorporating face oils into your routine can also enhance the benefits of these practices, providing a soothing aroma and nourishing the skin at the same time. Remember, taking care of your mind and body is essential for overall health and well-being.

Chapter 9. The Future of Face Yoga and Face Oils: Discussing the latest trends and developments in Face Yoga and face oils, and where the future of these practices may be headed.

Face Yoga and face oils have been gaining popularity in recent years, as people look for natural and effective ways to improve the health and appearance of their skin. As with any trend, there are always new developments and innovations on the horizon. In this chapter, we'll discuss the latest trends and developments in Face Yoga and face oils, and where the future of these practices may be headed.

The Rise of Technology

Technology has been making its way into the world of Face Yoga and face oils, with the rise of apps, online classes, and virtual consultations. Many Face Yoga instructors and skincare experts are now offering virtual classes and consultations, making it easier than ever to learn and practice Face Yoga and incorporate face oils into your skincare routine.

Innovations in Face Oils

As the popularity of face oils continues to grow, there are more and more options on the market. In addition to traditional oils such as jojoba, argan, and rosehip, there are now more specialized oils available, such as oils for specific skin concerns and oil blends for different times of day or seasons. As technology continues to advance, there may also be new ways to extract and process oils, leading to even more innovative and effective face oils.

Combining Face Yoga and Skincare

Face Yoga and skincare have always gone hand in hand, but in the future, we may see even more integration between the two. Some skincare brands are already incorporating Face Yoga exercises into their marketing and product offerings, with the goal of providing a holistic approach to skincare. As more people become aware of the benefits of Face Yoga, we may see even more collaboration between Face Yoga instructors and skincare brands.

Personalization and Customization

As with skincare, there is a growing trend towards personalization and customization in Face Yoga and face oils. More and more people are seeking out personalized recommendations for their skin concerns and goals, whether it be through virtual consultations or AI-powered skincare tools. In the future, we may see even more customized Face Yoga routines and face oil blends that are tailored to individual needs.

Conclusion

Face Yoga and face oils are here to stay, and as technology continues to advance and more people become aware of the benefits of these practices, we can expect to see even more innovations and developments in the future. Whether it's the integration of technology, the development of new oils and blends, or the increased personalization and customization of Face Yoga routines, the future of Face Yoga and face oils looks bright.

Chapter 10. Precautions and Safety Measures: Providing precautions and safety measures that should be taken when practicing Face Yoga and using face oils.

While Face Yoga and face oils can be effective ways to improve the health and appearance of your skin, it's important to take precautions and practice these techniques safely. In this chapter, we'll provide precautions and safety measures that should be taken when practicing Face Yoga and using face oils.

Precautions for Face Yoga:

1. **Avoid Overexertion:** While it's important to practice Face Yoga regularly to see the benefits, it's also important not to overexert your facial muscles. Start slowly and gradually increase the intensity of your exercises over time.

2. **Be Gentle:** Your facial skin is delicate and sensitive, so it's important to be gentle when practicing Face Yoga. Avoid pulling or tugging at the skin, and use light pressure when performing facial massage and acupressure.

3. **Listen to Your Body:** If you experience any pain or discomfort while practicing Face Yoga, stop immediately. It's important to listen to your body and take breaks when needed.

4. **Consult with Your Doctor:** If you have any medical conditions or concerns, it's important to consult with your doctor before practicing Face Yoga.

Precautions for Face Oils:

1. **Patch Test:** Before applying any new face oil to your skin, it's important to perform a patch test to ensure that you don't have an allergic reaction. Apply a small amount of the oil to your inner forearm and wait 24 hours to see if any redness or irritation occurs.

2. **Check the Ingredients:** Always check the ingredients of any face oil you plan to use to ensure that you are not allergic to any of the ingredients.

3. **Don't Overapply:** While face oils can be beneficial for the skin, it's important not to overapply them. Use a few drops of oil at a time and massage them into your skin using gentle upward strokes.

4. **Store Properly:** Face oils should be stored in a cool, dark place to prevent them from going rancid. Always check the expiration date and discard any oils that have gone bad.

Conclusion

By taking precautions and practicing Face Yoga and using face oils safely, you can enjoy the many benefits of these practices without any negative side effects. Remember to be gentle when practicing Face Yoga, listen to your body, and consult with your doctor if you have any concerns.

When using face oils, perform a patch test, check the ingredients, don't overapply, and store them properly. By following these precautions and safety measures, you can incorporate Face Yoga and face oils into your skincare routine with confidence.

Chapter 11. Combining Face Yoga and Face Oils with Other Skincare Practices: Discussing how Face Yoga and face oils can be used in conjunction with other skincare practices such as cleansing, toning, and exfoliating.

Face Yoga and face oils can be great additions to your skincare routine, but they can also be used in conjunction with other skincare practices such as cleansing, toning, and exfoliating to maximize their benefits. In this chapter, we'll discuss how you can combine Face Yoga and face oils with other skincare practices for optimal results.

Cleansing

Cleansing is an important step in any skincare routine, as it helps to remove dirt, oil, and impurities from the skin. When combining cleansing with Face Yoga and face oils, it's important to choose a gentle cleanser that won't strip the skin of its natural oils. After cleansing, you can apply a few drops of face oil to your fingertips and massage it into your skin using gentle upward strokes. This will help to nourish and protect your skin while also providing a slip for your fingers during Face Yoga exercises.

Toning

Toning is another important step in any skincare routine, as it helps to balance the pH of the skin and prepare it for the next steps in your routine. When combining toning with Face Yoga and face oils, it's important to choose a toner that is gentle and alcohol-free. After toning, you can apply a few drops of face oil to your fingertips and massage it into your skin using gentle upward strokes. This will help to nourish and protect your skin while also providing a slip for your fingers during Face Yoga exercises.

Exfoliating

Exfoliating is a key step in any skincare routine, as it helps to remove dead skin cells and promote cell turnover. When combining exfoliating with Face Yoga and face oils, it's important to choose an exfoliator that is gentle and suitable for your skin type. After exfoliating, you can apply a few drops of face oil to your fingertips and massage it into your skin using gentle upward strokes. This will help to nourish and protect your skin while also providing a slip for your fingers during Face Yoga exercises.

Conclusion

By combining Face Yoga and face oils with other skincare practices such as cleansing, toning, and exfoliating, you can maximize the benefits of these practices and achieve optimal results. Remember to choose gentle products that are suitable for your skin type, and always be gentle when performing Face Yoga exercises or massaging face oils into your skin. With a little patience and consistency, you can enjoy the many benefits of Face Yoga and face oils in conjunction with other skincare practices for healthy, glowing skin.

Chapter 12. Face Yoga and Face Oils for Different Skin Types: Providing guidelines for using Face Yoga and face oils for different skin types such as oily, dry, and sensitive skin.

Face Yoga and face oils can benefit all skin types, but it's important to use them in a way that is tailored to your specific skin type. In this chapter, we'll provide guidelines for using Face Yoga and face oils for different skin types, including oily, dry, and sensitive skin.

Oily Skin

If you have oily skin, you may be hesitant to use face oils, but they can be beneficial for balancing oil production and providing hydration without clogging pores. Look for lightweight face oils that absorb easily into the skin, such as jojoba or grapeseed oil. When practicing Face Yoga, focus on exercises that promote lymphatic drainage and improve circulation, such as facial massage and acupressure. Avoid using heavy creams or rich moisturizers that may contribute to excess oil production.

Dry Skin

If you have dry skin, face oils can be a game-changer, providing much-needed hydration and nourishment to the skin. Look for rich face oils that are packed with nourishing ingredients, such as argan or rosehip oil. When practicing Face Yoga, focus on exercises that promote hydration and stimulate collagen production, such as facial massage and facial exercises. Use a gentle cleanser and toner that won't strip the skin of its natural oils and consider adding a hydrating serum or moisturizer to your routine.

Sensitive Skin

If you have sensitive skin, it's important to use gentle, non-irritating products, including face oils and Face Yoga techniques. Look for face oils that are free of fragrances and harsh chemicals, such as chamomile or calendula oil. When practicing Face Yoga, focus on exercises that promote relaxation and reduce inflammation, such as facial massage and acupressure. Avoid using harsh exfoliants or scrubs and be gentle when massaging the skin.

Combination Skin

If you have combination skin, with both oily and dry areas, you'll need to balance hydration and oil production without causing irritation. Look for lightweight face oils that absorb easily into the skin, such as jojoba or argan oil. When practicing Face Yoga, focus on exercises that promote balance and harmony in the skin, such as facial massage and facial exercises. Use a gentle cleanser and toner that won't strip the skin of its natural oils and consider using a targeted serum or moisturizer for the dry areas of the skin.

Conclusion

By using Face Yoga and face oils in a way that is tailored to your specific skin type, you can maximize their benefits and achieve healthy, glowing skin. Remember to choose gentle, non-irritating products, and be gentle when performing Face Yoga exercises or massaging face oils into your skin. With a little patience and consistency, you can enjoy the many benefits of Face Yoga and face oils for your specific skin type.

Chapter 13. Success Stories and Testimonials: Sharing success stories and testimonials from individuals who have experienced positive results from incorporating Face Yoga and face oils into their skincare routine.

Face Yoga and face oils have gained popularity in recent years, with many individuals incorporating these practices into their skincare routine. In this chapter, we'll share success stories and testimonials from individuals who have experienced positive results from incorporating Face Yoga and face oils into their skincare routine.

Success Story #1: Jane

Jane, a 42-year-old mother of two, had been struggling with fine lines and wrinkles on her face. She tried various skincare products, but nothing seemed to work. Then, she discovered Face Yoga and face oils. After incorporating these practices into her skincare routine for a few weeks, she noticed a significant improvement in the texture and appearance of her skin. Her wrinkles were less noticeable, and her skin looked smoother and more radiant. She now swears by Face Yoga and face oils and recommends them to all her friends.

Success Story #2: Mike

Mike, a 35-year-old businessman, had been dealing with stress and anxiety, which was taking a toll on his skin. He had developed dark circles and puffiness under his eyes, and his skin looked dull and tired. After learning about Face Yoga and face oils, he decided to give them a try. He practiced facial massage and acupressure every day and incorporated a face oil into his skincare routine. Within a few weeks, he noticed a significant improvement in his skin. His dark circles and puffiness had reduced, and his skin looked brighter and more vibrant. He now practices Face Yoga and uses face oils regularly to maintain his healthy and glowing skin.

Testimonial #1: "I've been using face oils for years, but since incorporating Face Yoga into my skincare routine, I've noticed a significant improvement in the appearance of my skin. My wrinkles are less noticeable, and my skin looks more youthful and radiant. I'm so glad I discovered Face Yoga!" - Sarah, 50

Testimonial #2: "I was skeptical about Face Yoga at first, but after incorporating it into my daily routine, I've noticed a significant improvement in my skin's texture and tone. My skin looks smoother and more even, and my fine lines have reduced. I also love using face oils to hydrate and nourish my skin. I'll never go back to my old skincare routine!" - Emily, 32

Testimonial #3: "I have always had sensitive skin and struggled with finding skincare products that wouldn't irritate it. Since incorporating face oils into my routine, I have noticed a significant reduction in redness and irritation. And when I started practicing Face Yoga, I noticed a further improvement in the texture and appearance of my skin. It feels amazing to finally have found something that works for my skin!" - Michelle, 28

Success Story #3: Linda

Linda, a 60-year-old retiree, had been dealing with sagging skin and loss of firmness. She was considering invasive cosmetic procedures, but was hesitant due to the potential risks and side effects. Then, she discovered Face Yoga and face oils. She practiced facial exercises and acupressure regularly and incorporated a firming face oil into her routine. Within a few months, she noticed a significant improvement in the firmness and elasticity of her skin. Her sagging skin had lifted, and her skin looked more youthful and toned. She was thrilled with the results and decided to continue using Face Yoga and face oils to maintain her healthy and glowing skin.

Testimonial #4: "I was looking for a natural way to improve the health and appearance of my skin, and Face Yoga and face oils were the answer. After incorporating these practices into my skincare routine, I have noticed a significant improvement in my skin's hydration, texture, and radiance. I feel confident and beautiful in my own skin!" - Maria, 45

Conclusion

These success stories and testimonials are a testament to the power of Face Yoga and face oils in promoting healthy, radiant skin. Whether you're dealing with fine lines and wrinkles, dark circles and puffiness, or sagging skin and loss of firmness, these practices can help you achieve your skincare goals naturally and safely. So why not give them a try and see the positive results for yourself? With dedication and consistency, you can achieve beautiful, healthy, and glowing skin at any age.

Chapter 14. FAQs and Solutions: Addressing common questions and concerns related to Face Yoga and face oils and providing solutions for any issues that may arise.

Face Yoga and face oils have become increasingly popular in recent years, but with any new practice, there may be questions and concerns that arise. In this chapter, we'll address some common questions and concerns related to Face Yoga and face oils and provide troubleshooting solutions for any issues that may arise.

Frequently Asked Questions:

Q: Is Face Yoga suitable for all ages? A: Yes, Face Yoga is suitable for all ages, from teenagers to seniors. It can benefit individuals of all ages and skin types.

Q: How often should I practice Face Yoga? A: It is recommended to practice Face Yoga for at least 10-15 minutes a day, but you can do it for longer if you wish. Consistency is key, so try to incorporate it into your daily routine.

Q: Can Face Yoga help reduce the signs of aging? A: Yes, Face Yoga can help reduce the signs of aging by improving circulation, toning facial muscles, and promoting lymphatic drainage. It can also help to reduce the appearance of fine lines and wrinkles.

Q: Can face oils clog pores? A: Some face oils may clog pores, particularly if they are heavy or contain comedogenic ingredients. It's important to choose a lightweight face oil that is suitable for your skin type and won't clog your pores.

Q: Can face oils replace moisturizer? A: It depends on your skin type and the face oil you're using. Some face oils can be used as a moisturizer, particularly if they are rich and nourishing. However, if you have very dry skin, you may need to use a moisturizer in addition to a face oil.

Solutions:

Issue #1: My face oil feels too heavy on my skin. Solution: Try using a lighter face oil or applying a smaller amount. You can also try applying the face oil to damp skin, which can help it absorb better.

Issue #2: I'm not seeing any results from Face Yoga. Solution: It may take some time to see results from Face Yoga, so be patient and consistent with your practice. Make sure you're using proper technique and focusing on exercises that target your specific skincare concerns.

Issue #3: Face Yoga is causing me pain or discomfort. Solution: If you're experiencing pain or discomfort during Face Yoga, stop the exercise and try a gentler approach. Make sure you're not applying too much pressure, and adjust your technique as needed. You can also consult a Face Yoga instructor for guidance.

Issue #4: My face oil is causing breakouts. Solution: It's possible that your face oil is clogging your pores, so try switching to a lightweight oil that is non-comedogenic. Make sure you're not using too much oil, and avoid applying it to areas that are prone to breakouts.

Issue #5: I'm allergic to a particular face oil. Solution: If you're allergic to a particular face oil, discontinue use immediately and consult a dermatologist. They can help determine the cause of the allergic reaction and provide recommendations for suitable alternatives.

Issue #6: Face Yoga is taking too much time out of my day.
Solution: If you're finding it challenging to incorporate Face Yoga into your daily routine, try breaking it up into shorter sessions throughout the day. Even five minutes of Face Yoga can make a difference. You can also try multitasking by doing Face Yoga while watching TV or listening to music.

Issue #7: I'm not sure which face oil is suitable for my skin type.
Solution: Consult a skincare professional or dermatologist to determine which face oil is suitable for your skin type. They can also recommend other products that can complement your skincare routine, such as cleansers, toners, and serums.

Issue #8: I'm not comfortable performing Face Yoga in public.
Solution: You don't have to perform Face Yoga in public. You can do it in the privacy of your own home, or even incorporate it into your bedtime routine. You can also try doing Face Yoga in a private space, such as a restroom, if you're in a public setting.

Conclusion

By addressing these common issues and providing practical solutions, you can troubleshoot any problems that may arise when incorporating Face Yoga and face oils into your skincare routine. Remember, it's important to choose products that are suitable for your skin type and to be patient and consistent with your practice. With dedication and perseverance, you can achieve healthy, glowing skin through the power of Face Yoga and face oils.

Chapter 15. Face Yoga Exercises

Facial exercises, also known as Face Yoga, are a simple and effective way to improve the health and appearance of your skin. These exercises work by strengthening the muscles in your face, increasing blood flow, and reducing stress and tension.

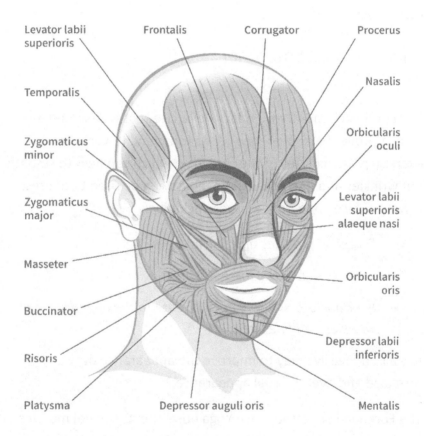

Over time, regular practice of Face Yoga can help to improve skin tone, reduce the appearance of wrinkles, and give your face a more youthful and radiant appearance.

There are over 43 muscles in the face. This chart displays some of these facial muscles.

In this chapter, we will provide a comprehensive guide to some of the most effective facial exercises. Whether you are looking to improve the overall health of your skin or simply want to reduce the appearance of fine lines and wrinkles, Face Yoga is a simple and effective solution that can be done from the comfort of your own home.

The Forehead Smoother

The Forehead Smoother is a facial exercise that is designed to help improve the appearance of the forehead. It works by exercising the muscles of the forehead, which can help to smooth out wrinkles and fine lines. This exercise can be used to address a variety of face appearance issues, including:

- *Forehead wrinkles and fine lines*

- *Sagging skin in the forehead area*

- *Poor posture, which can contribute to the appearance of wrinkles and fine lines*

It is a non-invasive way to improve the appearance of the forehead and overall facial appearance.

The Forehead Smoother Face Yoga pose affects several muscles in the forehead area, including:

1. **Frontalis muscle:** The frontalis muscle is a thin muscle that covers the forehead and is responsible for raising the eyebrows and creating forehead wrinkles.

2. **Corrugator supercilii muscle:** The corrugator supercilii muscle is a small muscle that runs from the eyebrow to the forehead and is responsible for pulling the eyebrows downward and inward, creating frown lines between the eyebrows.

3. **Orbicularis oculi muscle:** The orbicularis oculi muscle is a circular muscle around the eyes and is responsible for closing the eyelids and creating wrinkles around the eyes.

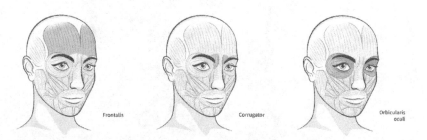

Frontalis   Corrugator   Orbicularis oculi

By pressing the palms into the forehead and sliding them upwards towards the hairline, The Forehead Smoother Face Yoga pose helps to stimulate blood flow to these muscles, relaxing them and reducing tension. This can help reduce the appearance of forehead wrinkles and frown lines, promoting a more youthful and relaxed appearance.

Here's how to do it:

Apply some facial oil to the palms of your hands and then massage it onto your face and neck, making sure to cover all areas where you will be performing Face Yoga exercises.

1. Sit or stand in a comfortable position with your back straight and shoulders relaxed.

2. Place your palms on your forehead with your fingertips facing each other.

3. Gently press your palms into your forehead and slide them upwards towards your hairline, using a smooth, sweeping motion.

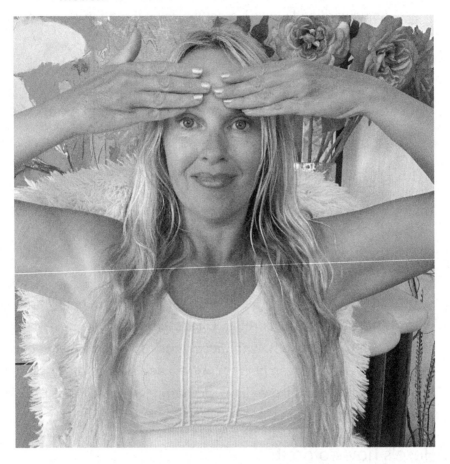

4. When you reach your hairline, release your palms and repeat the motion for a total of 10 to 15 repetitions.

5. Finish by placing your palms over your closed eyes and taking a few deep breaths.

This exercise helps to improve circulation in the forehead area and relaxes the muscles, which can help reduce the appearance of wrinkles and lines. It can be done daily as part of your skincare routine, or as needed throughout the day to relieve tension and stress in the forehead area. As with any exercise, it is important to start slowly and avoid any movements that cause discomfort or pain.

The Eye Firmer

The Eye Firmer is a facial exercise that is designed to help improve the appearance of the eyes. It works by exercising the muscles of the eyes, which can help to reduce the appearance of wrinkles and fine lines, as well as improve circulation in the area. This exercise can be used to address a variety of face appearance issues, including:

- *Crow's feet and other wrinkles around the eyes*

- *Dark circles and puffiness under the eyes*

- *Sagging skin in the eye area*

- *Poor circulation, which can contribute to the appearance of dark circles and puffiness under the eyes*

It is a non-invasive way to improve the appearance of the eyes and overall facial appearance.

The Eye Firmer Face Yoga pose targets the muscles around the eyes, including:

1. **Orbicularis oculi muscle:** The orbicularis oculi muscle is a circular muscle around the eyes and is responsible for closing the eyelids and creating wrinkles around the eyes.

2. **Corrugator supercilii muscle:** The corrugator supercilii muscle is a small muscle that runs from the eyebrow to the forehead and is responsible for pulling the eyebrows

downward and inward, creating frown lines between the eyebrows.

3. **Procerus muscle:** The procerus muscle is a small muscle between the eyebrows and is responsible for pulling the eyebrows downward and wrinkling the skin between them.

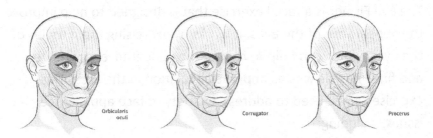

Orbicularis oculi Corrugator Procerus

By applying gentle pressure with the index fingers under the eyebrows and then squinting the eyes, The Eye Firmer Face Yoga pose helps to activate and tone these muscles, promoting a more lifted and toned appearance around the eyes. The repeated contraction and relaxation of these muscles can also help to increase blood flow and stimulate collagen production, reducing the appearance of fine lines and wrinkles.

The Eye Firmer aims to tone and strengthen the muscles around the eyes, reducing the appearance of crow's feet and fine lines.

Here's how to do it:

Apply some facial oil to the palms of your hands and then massage it onto your face and neck, making sure to cover all areas where you will be performing Face Yoga exercises.

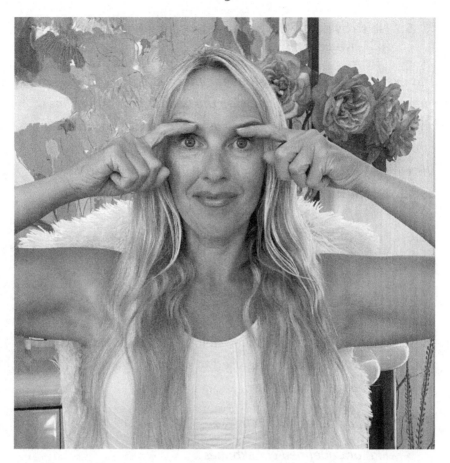

1. Sit or stand in a comfortable position with your back straight and shoulders relaxed.

2. Place your index fingers under your eyebrows, near the bridge of your nose.

3. Apply light pressure with your fingers and gently pull your skin upwards towards your hairline.

4. While holding this position, squint your eyes and then relax them. Repeat this squint and release movement for 10 to 15 repetitions.

5. Finish by gently massaging your temples and taking a few deep breaths.

This exercise helps to strengthen the muscles around the eyes, improving their tone and reducing the appearance of fine lines and wrinkles. It can be done daily as part of your skincare routine, or as needed throughout the day to relieve tension and stress in the eye area. As with any exercise, it is important to start slowly and avoid any movements that cause discomfort or pain.

The Cheek Lifter

The Cheek Lifter is a facial exercise that is designed to help improve the appearance of the cheeks. It works by exercising the muscles of the cheeks, which can help to lift and tone the skin in this area. This exercise can be used to address a variety of face appearance issues, including:

- *Sagging or drooping cheeks*

- *Flat or undefined cheekbones*

- *Poor posture, which can contribute to the appearance of sagging or drooping cheeks*

It is a non-invasive way to improve the appearance of the cheeks and overall facial appearance.

The Cheek Lifter targets the muscles in the cheek area, including:

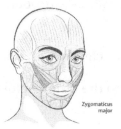
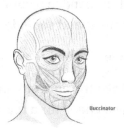

1. **Zygomaticus major muscle:** The zygomaticus major muscle is a facial muscle that extends from the cheekbone to the corners of the mouth and is responsible for smiling.

2. **Buccinator muscle:** The buccinator muscle is a thin, flat muscle in the cheek area that helps with chewing and smiling.

By filling the cheeks with air and moving the air from one cheek to the other, The Cheek Lifter Face Yoga pose helps to activate and tone these muscles, creating a more lifted and defined cheekbone area. The repeated contraction and relaxation of these muscles can also help to increase blood flow and stimulate collagen production, reducing the appearance of sagging and promoting a more youthful and radiant appearance.

The Cheek Lifter is a Face Yoga pose that aims to tone and lift the muscles in the cheeks, reducing sagging and creating a more defined cheekbone area.

Here's how to do it:

Apply some facial oil to the palms of your hands and then massage it onto your face and neck, making sure to cover all areas where you will be performing Face Yoga exercises.

1. Sit or stand in a comfortable position with your back straight and shoulders relaxed.

2. Take a deep breath and fill your cheeks with air.

3. Move the air from one cheek to the other, holding it in each cheek for a few seconds.

4. Exhale the air through your mouth and relax your facial muscles.

5. Repeat this exercise for 10 to 15 repetitions.

6. Finish by gently massaging your cheeks and taking a few deep breaths.

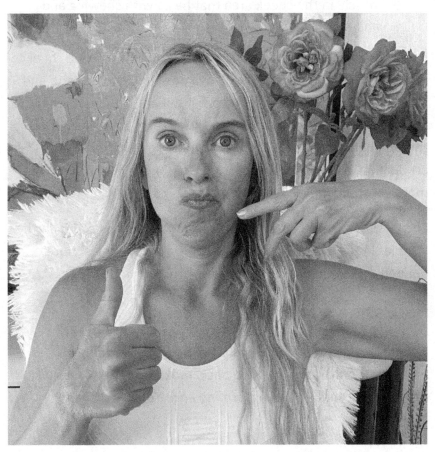

This exercise helps to strengthen and tone the muscles in the cheeks, creating a more defined and lifted cheekbone area. It can be done daily as part of your skincare routine, or as needed throughout the day to relieve tension and stress in the cheek area. As with any exercise, it is important to start slowly and avoid any movements that cause discomfort or pain. It is also important to maintain a proper diet and exercise regimen to help support overall skin health and vitality.

The Jaw Definer

The Jaw Definer is a facial exercise that is designed to help improve the appearance of the jawline. It works by exercising the muscles of the jaw, neck, and face, which can help to strengthen and define the jawline. This exercise can be used to address a variety of face appearance issues, including:

- *A weak or undefined jawline*

- *A double chin*

- *Sagging skin in the neck and jaw area*

- *Poor posture, which can make the face appear less defined*

It is a non-invasive way to improve the jawline and overall facial appearance.

The names of the muscles targeted by The Jaw Definer pose in Face Yoga are the masseter muscles and the platysma muscles.

1. **Masseter muscles:** These are the strongest muscles in the jaw and are responsible for moving the jaw during

chewing, talking, and other jaw-related movements. They are located on each side of the face, between the cheekbone and the lower jawbone.

2. **Platysma muscles:** These muscles run from the collarbone and shoulder region up to the lower face and jawline. They help to support the lower face and jaw and are also involved in facial expressions like frowning and grimacing.

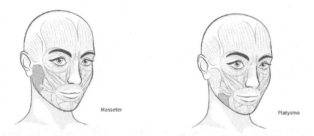

By targeting and strengthening these muscles through Face Yoga exercises like The Jaw Definer pose, you can help to tone and define the jawline, reduce sagging or drooping in the lower face and neck, and improve overall facial symmetry and balance.

Here's how to do it:

Apply some facial oil to the palms of your hands and then massage it onto your face and neck, making sure to cover all areas where you will be performing Face Yoga exercises.

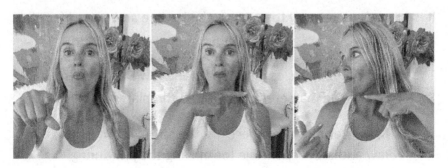

1. Begin by sitting or standing up straight with your head facing forward.

2. Relax your shoulders and take a few deep breaths.

3. Slowly begin to open your mouth as wide as you can, while keeping your lips together and your teeth slightly apart.

4. Next, move your lower jaw forward and back, as if you were chewing, for 20-30 seconds.

5. Then, move your jaw to the right and hold for 5-10 seconds. Repeat on the left side.

6. Finally, relax your jaw and return to a neutral position.

Repeat this exercise 5-10 times, or as many times as you feel comfortable. Over time, you may notice a more defined and toned jawline.

The Chin Tuck

The Chin Tuck is a facial exercise that is designed to help improve the appearance of the chin and neck. It works by exercising the muscles of the chin and neck, which can help to strengthen and tone the skin in this area. This exercise can be used to address a variety of face appearance issues, including:

- *A weak or undefined chin*

- *A double chin*

- *Sagging skin in the neck and chin area*

- *Poor posture, which can make the face appear less defined*

It is a non-invasive way to improve the appearance of the chin and neck and overall facial appearance.

The Chin Tuck primarily targets the muscles in the neck and upper back, which help to support the head and maintain good posture. Specifically, The Chin Tuck can help to strengthen the deep cervical flexors, which are the muscles that run along the front of the neck and help to stabilize the head and neck. These muscles are often weakened by poor posture, which can lead to neck pain, headaches, and other issues.

In addition to the deep cervical flexors, The Chin Tuck can also engage the muscles in the jaw and throat, which can help to improve facial symmetry and reduce tension in the face and neck. This can be particularly beneficial for those who spend long hours working at a computer or looking down at a smartphone, as it can help to counteract the effects of "tech neck" and promote better alignment and circulation throughout the body.

The muscles that are primarily targeted during The Chin Tuck are the deep cervical flexors, which include the following muscles:

1. Longus capitis

2. Longus colli

3. Rectus capitis anterior

4. Rectus capitis lateralis

5. Rectus capitis posterior minor

6. Rectus capitis posterior major

7. Obliquus capitis superior

8. Obliquus capitis inferior

These muscles work together to support the head and neck, and help to maintain proper posture and alignment. When these muscles become weak or imbalanced, it can lead to issues such as neck pain, headaches, and poor posture. Practicing The Chin Tuck pose can help to strengthen these muscles and improve overall neck and spine health.

Here's how to do it:

Apply some facial oil to the palms of your hands and then massage it onto your face and neck, making sure to cover all areas where you will be performing Face Yoga exercises.

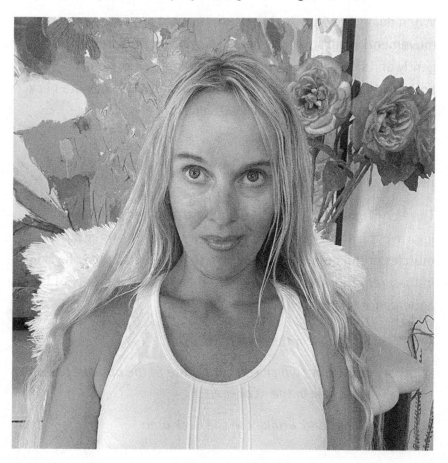

1. Begin by sitting or standing tall with your shoulders relaxed and your spine elongated.

2. Gently tilt your chin down towards your chest, as if you're nodding your head.

3. Keep your gaze forward and focus on lengthening the back of your neck.

4. Hold the position for a few breaths, and then release.

5. Repeat several times, gradually increasing the duration of each hold.

When doing The Chin Tuck, be sure to avoid any excessive movements or strain in the neck. This pose should be performed gently and slowly, with a focus on proper alignment and breathing. Over time, it can help improve posture, alleviate neck tension, and enhance overall well-being.

The Neck Tightener

The Neck Tightener is a facial exercise that is designed to help improve the appearance of the neck. It works by exercising the muscles of the neck, which can help to tighten and tone the skin in this area. This exercise can be used to address a variety of face appearance issues, including:

- *Sagging skin in the neck area*

- *Poor posture, which can contribute to the appearance of sagging skin in the neck area*

- *Fine lines and wrinkles in the neck area*

- *"Tech neck", which is characterized by a forward-leaning head and neck position and can result in the development of wrinkles and fine lines in the neck and jaw area*

It is a non-invasive way to improve the appearance of the neck and overall facial appearance.

This exercise targets the muscles in the neck and jaw, helping to improve their strength and tone. It can also help to promote better circulation in the face and neck and may help reduce the appearance of wrinkles or sagging skin in these areas.

1. **Sternocleidomastoid (SCM) muscle:** This muscle runs from the base of the skull to the collarbone and is responsible for turning and tilting the head. When the head is tilted back in the exercise, the SCM muscle is engaged.

2. **Platysma muscle:** This muscle runs from the chin to the collarbone and helps to lift the chin and corners of the mouth. When the tongue is pressed against the roof of the mouth in the exercise, the platysma muscle is activated.

3. **Hyoid muscles:** The hyoid bone is a small bone in the neck that supports the tongue and helps with swallowing. The exercise can help to engage the muscles around the hyoid bone, including the mylohyoid, geniohyoid, and digastric muscles.

By practicing this exercise regularly, you can help to tone and strengthen these muscles, which can help to improve the appearance of the neck and jawline and may also help to alleviate tension and stiffness in the neck. As always, it's important to practice this exercise with care and stop if you experience any discomfort or pain.

Here's how to do it:

Apply some facial oil to the palms of your hands and then massage it onto your face and neck, making sure to cover all areas where you will be performing Face Yoga exercises.

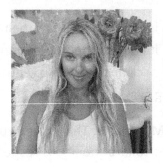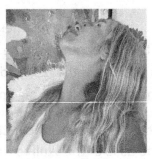

1. Begin by sitting or standing up straight with your shoulders relaxed and your neck elongated.

2. Tilt your head back and look up at the ceiling.

3. Press your tongue against the roof of your mouth and hold it there.

4. Slowly lower your chin towards your chest, while keeping your tongue pressed against the roof of your mouth.

5. Hold the position for a few seconds, then slowly lift your head back up to the starting position.

6. Repeat this exercise several times, gradually increasing the duration of each hold.

This exercise targets the muscles in the neck and jaw, helping to improve their strength and tone. It can also help to promote better circulation in the face and neck and may help reduce the appearance of wrinkles or sagging skin in these areas.

The Mouth Firmer

The Mouth Firmer is a facial exercise that is designed to help improve the appearance of the mouth and surrounding area. It works by exercising the muscles of the mouth and cheek, which can help to tighten and tone the skin in this area. This exercise can be used to address a variety of face appearance issues, including:

- *Sagging skin around the mouth*

- *Fine lines and wrinkles around the mouth and cheek area*

- *Poor posture, which can contribute to the appearance of sagging skin and fine lines*

It is a non-invasive way to improve the appearance of the mouth and surrounding area and overall facial appearance.

This pose can help to tone and strengthen these muscles, which can contribute to a firmer, more defined facial appearance.

Here are some of the muscles that The Mouth Firmer can affect:

1. **Orbicularis oris:** This is the circular muscle around the mouth that is responsible for puckering the lips and closing the mouth. The Mouth Firmer can help to engage and tone this muscle.

2. **Zygomaticus major and minor:** These muscles run from the cheekbones to the corners of the mouth and help to lift the cheeks and form a smile. The Mouth Firmer can help to activate and strengthen these muscles.

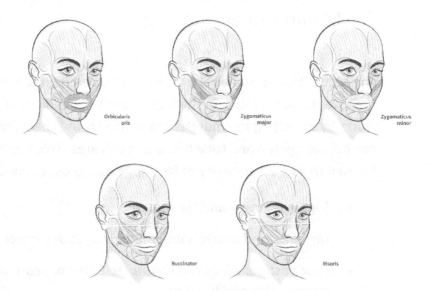

Orbicularis oris Zygomaticus major Zygomaticus minor Buccinator Risoris

3. **Buccinator:** This is a thin muscle in the cheeks that helps to compress the cheeks and push air out of the mouth. The Mouth Firmer can help to engage and tone this muscle.

4. **Risorius:** This is a narrow muscle that runs from the corners of the mouth to the cheeks. It helps to pull the corners of the mouth outwards and upwards, creating a smile. The Mouth Firmer can help to activate and tone this muscle.

By practicing The Mouth Firmer regularly, you can help to improve the strength and tone of these muscles, which can help to reduce the appearance of sagging skin, wrinkles, or fine lines around the mouth and cheeks. As with any exercise, it's important to practice The Mouth Firmer with care and stop if you experience any discomfort or pain.

Here's how to do it:

Apply some facial oil to the palms of your hands and then massage it onto your face and neck, making sure to cover all areas where you will be performing Face Yoga exercises.

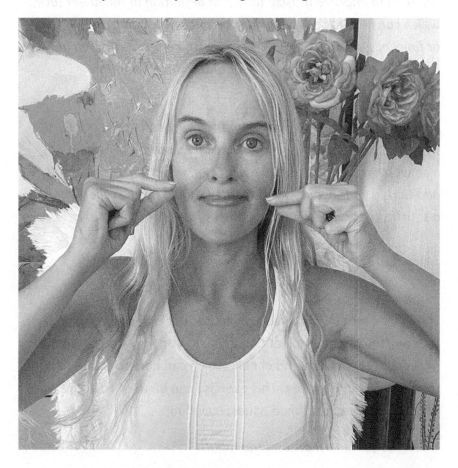

1. Begin by sitting or standing up straight with your shoulders relaxed.

2. Close your mouth and press your lips together tightly.

3. Hold the position for a few seconds, then release.

4. Repeat the exercise several times, gradually increasing the duration of each hold.

When doing the Mouth Firmer, you should feel a tightening sensation in the muscles around your mouth and cheeks. This pose can help to improve muscle tone and definition in the lower face, which can help to reduce the appearance of sagging skin, wrinkles, or fine lines. It may also help to promote better circulation in the face, which can contribute to a brighter, more youthful complexion.

As with any exercise, it's important to practice The Mouth Firmer with care and stop if you experience any discomfort or pain. It's also worth noting that while facial yoga poses can be a helpful addition to your beauty routine, they should not be relied upon as a substitute for a healthy lifestyle or professional skincare.

The Smile Smoother

The Smile Smoother is a facial exercise that is designed to help improve the appearance of the smile. It works by exercising the muscles of the mouth and cheek, which can help to tighten and tone the skin in this area. This exercise can be used to address a variety of face appearance issues, including:

- *Sagging skin around the mouth*

- *Fine lines and wrinkles around the mouth and cheek area*

- *Poor posture, which can contribute to the appearance of sagging skin and fine lines*

It is a non-invasive way to improve the appearance of the smile and overall facial appearance. It can help reduce tension and smooth out wrinkles around the mouth and cheeks.

This pose primarily targets the muscles around the mouth and cheeks. It can help to reduce tension and smooth out wrinkles in these areas.

Here are some of the muscles that The Smile Smoother can affect:

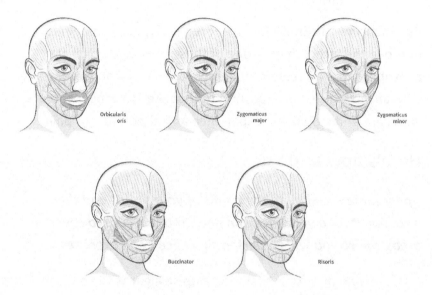

1. **Orbicularis oris:** This is the circular muscle around the mouth that is responsible for puckering the lips and closing the mouth. The Smile Smoother can help to activate and tone this muscle, as well as the muscles around the corners of the mouth.

2. **Zygomaticus major and minor:** These muscles run from the cheekbones to the corners of the mouth and help to lift the cheeks and form a smile. The Smile Smoother can help to activate and tone these muscles.

3. **Buccinator:** This is a thin muscle in the cheeks that helps to compress the cheeks and push air out of the mouth.

The Smile Smoother can help to engage and tone this muscle.

4. **Risorius:** This is a narrow muscle that runs from the corners of the mouth to the cheeks. It helps to pull the corners of the mouth outwards and upwards, creating a smile. The Smile Smoother can help to activate and tone this muscle.

By practicing The Smile Smoother regularly, you can help to improve the strength and tone of these muscles, which can contribute to a more youthful and relaxed facial appearance. As with any exercise, it's important to practice The Smile Smoother with care and stop if you experience any discomfort or pain.

Here's how to do it:

Apply some facial oil to the palms of your hands and then massage it onto your face and neck, making sure to cover all areas where you will be performing Face Yoga exercises.

1. Begin by sitting or standing up straight with your shoulders relaxed.

2. Place your index fingers on the corners of your mouth, with the rest of your fingers resting on your cheeks.

3. Gently pull the corners of your mouth back towards your ears.

4. While holding the position, try to smile as widely as you can without moving your fingers.

5. Hold the pose for a few seconds, then release.

6. Repeat the exercise several times, gradually increasing the duration of each hold.

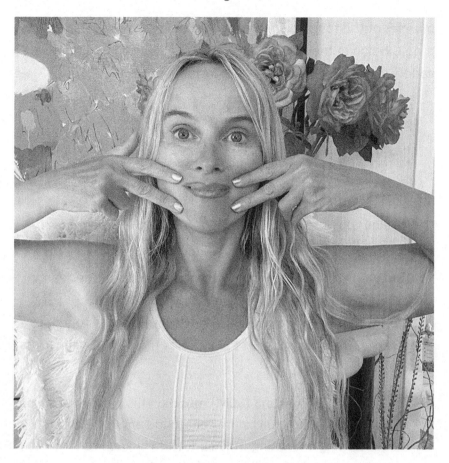

When doing the Smile Smoother, you should feel a gentle stretching sensation around your mouth and cheeks. This pose can help to reduce tension in the facial muscles. Muscle tension can contribute to the formation of wrinkles or fine lines. The Smile Smoother may also help to improve muscle tone and definition in the lower face, creating a more youthful and relaxed appearance.

The Tongue Press

The Tongue Press is a facial exercise that is designed to help improve the appearance of the face. It works by exercising the muscles of the tongue, which can help to improve circulation and tone the skin in the face. This exercise can be used to address a variety of face appearance issues, including:

- *Poor circulation, which can contribute to the appearance of dark circles and puffiness under the eyes*

- *Fine lines and wrinkles in the face*

- *Sagging skin in the face*

- *Poor posture, which can contribute to the appearance of fine lines and wrinkles*

The Tongue Press primarily targets the muscles in the neck and jaw area. This pose can help to tone and strengthen these muscles, which can contribute to a more youthful and toned appearance. Here are some of the muscles that The Tongue Press can affect:

1. **Sternocleidomastoid (SCM) muscle:** This muscle runs from the base of the skull to the collarbone and is responsible for turning and tilting the head. The Tongue Press can help to engage and tone this muscle.

2. **Hyoid muscles:** The hyoid bone is a small bone in the neck that supports the tongue and helps with swallowing. The Tongue Press can help to engage and tone the muscles around the hyoid bone, including the mylohyoid, geniohyoid, and digastric muscles.

3. **Muscles of mastication:** These are the muscles that are responsible for chewing and moving the jaw. The Tongue Press can help to engage and tone these muscles, which can contribute to a more defined and toned jawline.

By practicing The Tongue Press regularly, you can help to improve the strength and tone of these muscles, which can contribute to a more youthful and toned appearance in the neck and jaw area.

Here's how to do it:

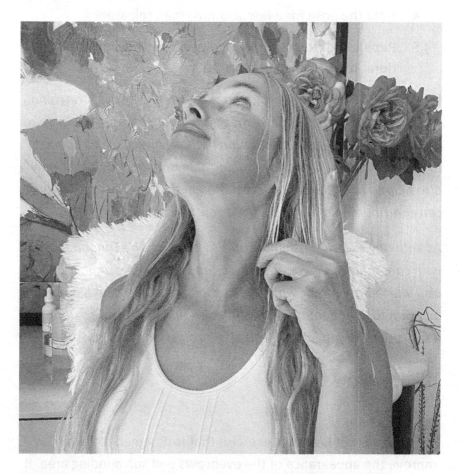

Apply some facial oil to the palms of your hands and then massage it onto your face and neck, making sure to cover all areas where you will be performing Face Yoga exercises.

1. Begin by sitting or standing up straight with your shoulders relaxed.

2. Press your tongue against the roof of your mouth with gentle pressure.

3. Slowly tilt your head back and look up towards the ceiling.

4. Hold the pose for a few seconds, then release.

5. Repeat the exercise several times, gradually increasing the duration of each hold.

When doing the Tongue Press, you should feel a gentle stretching sensation in the muscles of the neck and jaw. This pose can help to improve muscle tone and definition in these areas, which can help to reduce the appearance of sagging skin or a double chin. It may also help to promote better circulation in the face and neck, which can contribute to a brighter, more youthful complexion.

As with any exercise, it's important to practice The Tongue Press with care and stop if you experience any discomfort or pain. It's also worth noting that while facial yoga poses can be a helpful addition to your beauty routine, they should not be relied upon as a substitute for a healthy lifestyle or professional skincare.

The Eyebrow Lift

The Eyebrow Lift is a facial exercise that is designed to help improve the appearance of the eyebrows and surrounding area. It works by exercising the muscles of the forehead and brow, which can help to lift and tone the skin in this area. This exercise can be used to address a variety of face appearance issues, including:

- *Sagging skin in the forehead and brow area*

- *Fine lines and wrinkles in the forehead and brow area*

- *Poor posture, which can contribute to the appearance of fine lines and wrinkles*

The Eyebrow Lift primarily targets the muscles in the forehead and eye area. This pose can help to tone and lift these muscles, which can contribute to a more youthful and lifted appearance.

Here are some of the muscles that The Eyebrow Lift can affect:

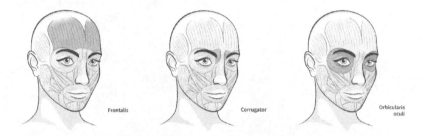

Frontalis   Corrugator   Orbicularis oculi

1. **Frontalis muscle:** This is a muscle that covers the forehead and helps to raise the eyebrows. The Eyebrow Lift can help to engage and tone this muscle.

2. **Corrugator supercilii muscle:** This muscle runs from the eyebrow to the bridge of the nose and helps to pull the eyebrows downwards. The Eyebrow Lift can help to counteract the downward pull of this muscle, leading to a more lifted appearance.

3. **Orbicularis oculi muscle:** This muscle surrounds the eye and is responsible for closing the eyelids. The Eyebrow Lift can help to engage and tone the muscles in this area, which can contribute to a brighter, more youthful appearance.

Here's how to do it:

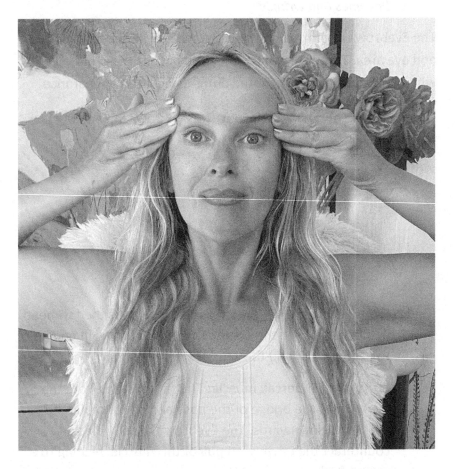

Apply some facial oil to the palms of your hands and then massage it onto your face and neck, making sure to cover all areas where you will be performing Face Yoga exercises.

1. Begin by sitting or standing up straight with your shoulders relaxed.

2. Place your fingertips at the outer corners of your eyebrows.

3. Gently lift your eyebrows upwards, using your fingertips to provide gentle resistance.

4. Hold the pose for a few seconds, then release.

5. Repeat the exercise several times, gradually increasing the duration of each hold.

When doing the Eyebrow Lift, you should feel a gentle stretching sensation in the muscles around the forehead and eyes. This pose can help to improve muscle tone and definition in these areas, which can contribute to a more youthful and lifted appearance. It may also help to reduce tension in the forehead and alleviate headaches or eyestrain.

As with any exercise, it's important to practice The Eyebrow Lift with care and stop if you experience any discomfort or pain. It's also worth noting that while facial yoga poses can be a helpful addition to your beauty routine, they should not be relied upon as a substitute for a healthy lifestyle or professional skincare.

The Nose Shaper

The Nose Shaper is a facial exercise that is designed to help improve the appearance of the nose. It works by exercising the muscles of the nose and surrounding area, which can help to tone and shape the skin in this area. This exercise can be used to address a variety of face appearance issues, including:

- *A flat or undefined nose*

- *Poor posture, which can contribute to the appearance of a flat or undefined nose*

- *Fine lines and wrinkles in the nose and surrounding area*

- *Sagging skin in the nose and surrounding area*

The Nose Shaper primarily targets the muscles around the nose and mouth. This pose can help to tone and strengthen these muscles, which can contribute to a more sculpted and defined facial appearance.

Here are some of the muscles that The Nose Shaper can affect:

1. **Nasalis muscle:** This is a paired muscle that runs from the nose to the upper lip and is responsible for flaring the nostrils. The Nose Shaper can help to engage and tone this muscle.

2. **Levator labii superioris alaeque nasi muscle:** This muscle runs from the upper lip to the nose and is responsible for lifting the upper lip and flaring the nostrils. The Nose Shaper can help to engage and tone this muscle.

3. **Depressor septi nasi muscle:** This muscle runs from the base of the nose to the upper lip and is responsible for pulling the nose downwards. The Nose Shaper can help to engage and tone this muscle.

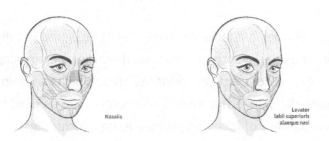

Nasalis

Levator
labii superioris
alaeque nasi

Here's how to do it:

Apply some facial oil to the palms of your hands and then massage it onto your face and neck, making sure to cover all

areas where you will be performing Face Yoga exercises.

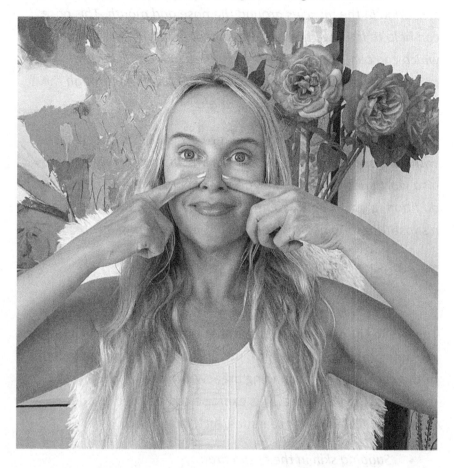

1. Begin by sitting or standing up straight with your shoulders relaxed.

2. Using your index fingers, press down on the sides of your nose, just above the nostrils.

3. While keeping your fingers in place, flare your nostrils and pull them downwards.

4. Hold the pose for a few seconds, then release.

5. Repeat the exercise several times, gradually increasing the duration of each hold.

When doing the Nose Shaper, you should feel a gentle stretching sensation in the muscles around the nose and mouth. This pose can help to improve muscle tone and definition in these areas, which can contribute to a more sculpted and defined facial appearance. It may also help to improve breathing through the nostrils and alleviate sinus congestion.

As with any exercise, it's important to practice The Nose Shaper with care and stop if you experience any discomfort or pain. It's also worth noting that while facial yoga poses can be a helpful addition to your beauty routine, they should not be relied upon as a substitute for a healthy lifestyle or professional skincare.

The Eyelid Lift

The Eyelid Lift is a facial exercise that is designed to help improve the appearance of the eyelids. It works by exercising the muscles of the eyelids and surrounding area, which can help to lift and tone the skin in this area. This exercise can be used to address a variety of face appearance issues, including:

- *Sagging skin in the eyelid area*

- *Fine lines and wrinkles in the eyelid area*

- *Poor posture, which can contribute to the appearance of fine lines and wrinkles*

It is a non-invasive way to improve the appearance of the eyelids and overall facial appearance.

The Eyelid Lift can help tone and lift the muscles around the eyes. It primarily targets the muscles around the eyes and forehead. This pose can help to tone and lift these muscles, which can contribute to a more youthful and lifted appearance.

Here are some of the muscles that The Eyelid Lift can affect:

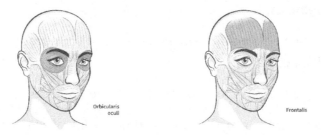

Orbicularis
oculi

Frontalis

1. **Levator palpebrae superioris muscle: This** muscle runs from the upper eyelid to the eyebrow and is responsible for lifting the upper eyelid. The Eyelid Lift can help to engage and tone this muscle.

2. **Orbicularis oculi muscle: This** muscle surrounds the eye and is responsible for closing the eyelids. The Eyelid Lift can help to engage and tone the muscles in this area, which can contribute to a brighter, more youthful appearance.

3. **Frontalis muscle:** This is a thin muscle that covers the forehead and helps to raise the eyebrows. The Eyelid Lift can help to engage and tone this muscle, which can help to reduce the appearance of wrinkles in the forehead area.

Here's how to do it:

Apply some facial oil to the palms of your hands and then massage it onto your face and neck, making sure to cover all areas where you will be performing Face Yoga exercises.

1. Begin by sitting or standing up straight with your shoulders relaxed.

2. Place your index fingers on the outer corners of your eyes, just above the eyebrows.

3. Gently pull the skin upwards and outwards towards your temples.

4. While holding the skin in place, open your eyes wide and look upwards.

5. Hold the pose for a few seconds, then release.

6. Repeat the exercise several times, gradually increasing the duration of each hold.

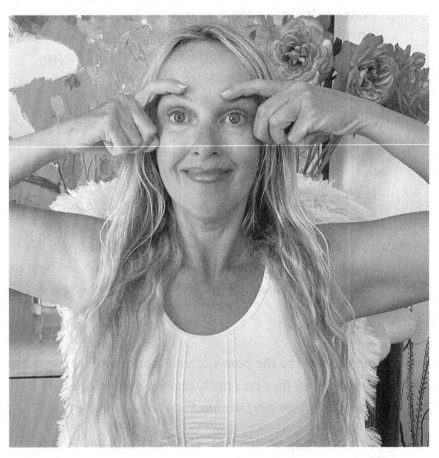

When doing The Eyelid Lift, you should feel a gentle stretching

sensation in the muscles around the eyes. This pose can help to improve muscle tone and definition in these areas, which can contribute to a more youthful and lifted appearance. It may also help to reduce tension in the forehead and alleviate headaches or eyestrain.

As with any exercise, it's important to practice The Eyelid Lift with care and stop if you experience any discomfort or pain. It's also worth noting that while facial yoga poses can be a helpful addition to your beauty routine, they should not be relied upon as a substitute for a healthy lifestyle or professional skincare.

The Lip Stretcher

The Lip Stretcher is a facial exercise that is designed to help improve the appearance of the lips and surrounding area. It works by exercising the muscles of the lips and cheek, which can help to tighten and tone the skin in this area. This exercise can be used to address a variety of face appearance issues, including:

- *Sagging skin around the mouth*

- *Fine lines and wrinkles around the mouth and cheek area*

- *Poor posture, which can contribute to the appearance of fine lines and wrinkles*

It is a non-invasive way to improve the appearance of the lips and surrounding area and overall facial appearance. This exercise can help tone and strengthen the muscles around the mouth and cheeks.

The Lip Stretcher can help to tone and strengthen these muscles, which can contribute to a more youthful and toned facial appearance. Here are some of the muscles that The Lip Stretcher can affect:

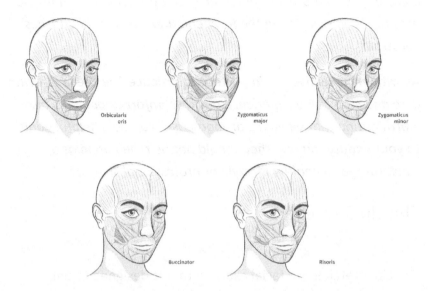

1. **Orbicularis oris muscle:** This is the circular muscle around the mouth that is responsible for puckering the lips and closing the mouth. The Lip Stretcher can help to engage and tone this muscle, as well as the muscles around the corners of the mouth.

2. **Zygomaticus major and minor muscles:** These muscles run from the cheekbones to the corners of the mouth and help to lift the cheeks and form a smile. The Lip Stretcher can help to engage and tone these muscles.

3. **Buccinator muscle:** This is a thin muscle in the cheeks that helps to compress the cheeks and push air out of the mouth. The Lip Stretcher can help to engage and tone this muscle.

4. **Risorius muscle:** This is a narrow muscle that runs from the corners of the mouth to the cheeks. It helps to pull the

corners of the mouth outwards and upwards, creating a smile. The Lip Stretcher can help to engage and tone this muscle.

Here's how to do it:

Apply some facial oil to the palms of your hands and then massage it onto your face and neck, making sure to cover all areas where you will be performing Face Yoga exercises.

1. Begin by sitting or standing up straight with your shoulders relaxed.

2. Open your mouth wide, as if you were yawning.

3. Place your index fingers on the corners of your mouth, with the rest of your fingers resting on your cheeks.

4. Gently pull the corners of your mouth outwards towards your ears.

5. While holding the position, try to smile as widely as you can without moving your fingers.

6. Hold the pose for a few seconds, then release.

Repeat the exercise several times, gradually increasing the duration of each hold.

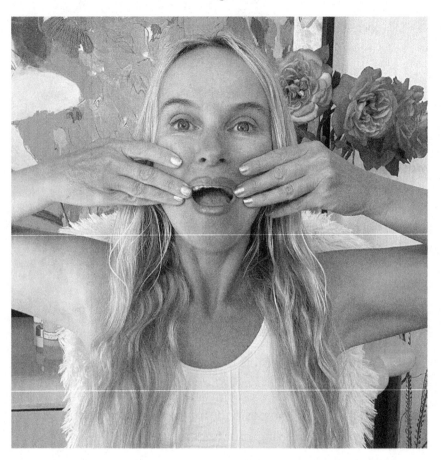

When doing The Lip Stretcher, you should feel a gentle stretching sensation around your mouth and cheeks. This pose can help to improve muscle tone and definition in these areas, which can contribute to a more youthful and toned facial appearance. It may also help to reduce tension in the facial muscles and improve circulation in the face.

The Fish Face

The Fish Face, also known as the "Blowing Fish Face Pose", is a facial exercise that is designed to help improve the appearance of the cheeks, jaw, and neck. It works by exercising the muscles of the cheeks, jaw, and neck, which can help to tighten and tone the skin in this area. This exercise can be used to address a variety of face appearance issues, including:

- *Sagging skin in the cheeks, jaw, and neck area*

- *Poor posture, which can contribute to the appearance of sagging skin*

- *Fine lines and wrinkles in the cheeks, jaw, and neck area*

- *A weak or undefined jawline*

The Fish Face pose, also known as the "Suck in Cheeks" pose, is a facial yoga exercise that primarily targets the muscles in the cheeks and lips. The main muscles targeted by this pose are the zygomaticus major and minor muscles, which are located in the cheek area and are responsible for elevating the corners of the mouth and creating a smile.

The Fish Face pose also targets the orbicularis oris muscle, which encircles the mouth and is responsible for puckering the lips. This exercise can help to tone and strengthen these muscles, which can help to improve the overall appearance of the face and reduce the appearance of wrinkles and fine lines around the mouth and cheek area.

The primary muscles targeted by this pose are the following:

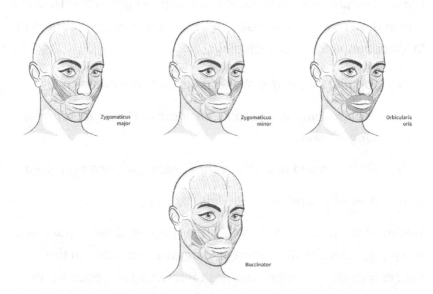

1. **Zygomaticus major muscle:** This muscle is located in the cheek area and extends from the zygomatic bone to the corner of the mouth. Its main function is to elevate the corners of the mouth, which creates a smile.

2. **Zygomaticus minor muscle:** This muscle is also located in the cheek area and is smaller than the zygomaticus major. Its function is similar to the zygomaticus major muscle and it also helps to elevate the corners of the mouth.

3. **Orbicularis oris muscle:** This muscle is a circular muscle that encircles the mouth and is responsible for closing and puckering the lips.

4. **Buccinator muscle:** This muscle is located in the cheek area and helps to compress the cheeks inward, which can create a more defined cheekbone appearance.

By performing The Fish Face pose, you can help to tone and

strengthen these muscles, which can improve the overall appearance of the face and reduce the appearance of wrinkles and fine lines in the cheek and mouth area.

Here's how to do it:

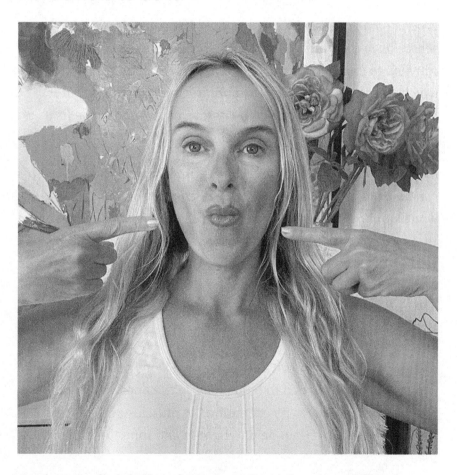

Apply some facial oil to the palms of your hands and then massage it onto your face and neck, making sure to cover all areas where you will be performing Face Yoga exercises.

1. Begin by sitting or standing up straight with your shoulders relaxed.

2. Suck in your cheeks and lips to make a "fish face" shape.

3. Hold the pose for a few seconds, then release.

4. Repeat the exercise several times, gradually increasing the duration of each hold.

When doing The Fish Face, you should feel a gentle stretching sensation in the muscles around the cheeks and jawline. This pose can help to improve muscle tone and definition in these areas, which can contribute to a more youthful and sculpted facial appearance. It may also help to improve circulation in the face and reduce tension in the facial muscles.

As with any exercise, it's important to practice The Fish Face with care and stop if you experience any discomfort or pain. It's also worth noting that while facial yoga poses can be a helpful addition to your beauty routine, they should not be relied upon as a substitute for a healthy lifestyle or professional skincare.

The Lion Face

The Lion Face, also known as the "Roaring Lion Pose", is a facial exercise that is designed to help improve the appearance of the face and neck. It works by exercising the muscles of the face, neck, and jaw, which can help to tighten and tone the skin in this area.

This exercise can be used to address a variety of face appearance issues, including:

- *Sagging skin in the face and neck area*

- *Poor posture, which can contribute to the appearance of sagging skin*

- *Fine lines and wrinkles in the face and neck area*

- *A weak or undefined jawline*

- *A double chin*

The Lion Face targets several muscles in the face and neck, including:

1. **Platysma muscle:** This muscle is located in the neck and helps to lift the jaw and lower lip.

2. **Sternocleidomastoid muscle:** This muscle is located in the neck and helps to turn the head and neck.

3. **Muscles around the mouth:** The Lion Face pose can also help to tone and strengthen the muscles around the mouth, including the orbicularis oris and the buccinator muscles.

Here's how to do it:

Apply some facial oil to the palms of your hands and then massage it onto your face and neck, making sure to cover all areas where you will be performing Face Yoga exercises.

1. Sit comfortably in a cross-legged position on the floor or a chair, with your back straight and your shoulders relaxed.

2. Inhale deeply through your nose, and as you exhale, open your mouth wide and stick out your tongue as far as you can, while simultaneously opening your eyes wide.

3. Contract the muscles in your throat and neck, and exhale while making a "ha" sound.

Repeat this exercise several times, taking deep breaths in between each repetition.

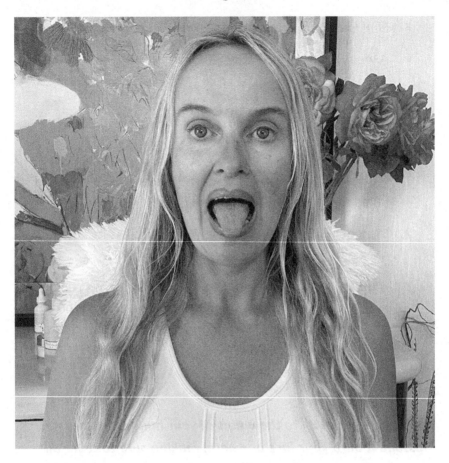

By performing The Lion Face pose regularly, you can help to improve the overall appearance of your face and reduce the appearance of wrinkles and fine lines in the face and neck area. Additionally, this pose can help to relieve tension in the neck and shoulders and promote relaxation.

The Forehead Wrinkle Smoother

The Forehead Wrinkle Smoother is a facial exercise that is

designed to help improve the appearance of the forehead and surrounding area. It works by exercising the muscles of the forehead, which can help to smooth and reduce the appearance of fine lines and wrinkles in this area. This exercise can be used to address a variety of face appearance issues, including:

- *Fine lines and wrinkles in the forehead and surrounding area*

- *Sagging skin in the forehead and surrounding area*

- *Poor posture, which can contribute to the appearance of fine lines and wrinkles*

This pose primarily targets the frontalis muscle, which is located in the forehead and is responsible for raising the eyebrows and creating wrinkles on the forehead.

When performing The Forehead Wrinkle Smoother, you place your fingers on your forehead and apply gentle pressure while moving the eyebrows up and down. This helps to strengthen and tone the frontalis muscle and improve blood circulation to the area, which can help reduce the appearance of wrinkles on the forehead over time.

In addition to **the frontalis muscle**, this pose may also engage other muscles in the face, including **the corrugator muscles**, which are responsible for creating vertical lines between the eyebrows, and the **orbicularis oculi muscles**, which are responsible for closing the eyes tightly. By engaging these muscles and promoting relaxation, The Forehead Wrinkle Smoother may help improve overall facial muscle tone and promote a more youthful appearance.

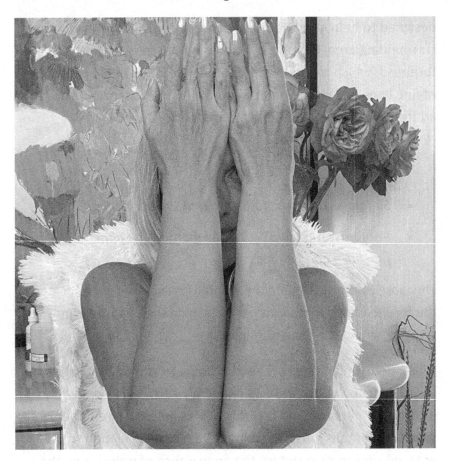

Here's how to do it:

Apply some facial oil to the palms of your hands and then massage it onto your face and neck, making sure to cover all areas where you will be performing Face Yoga exercises.

1. Sit comfortably in a cross-legged position on the floor or a chair, with your back straight and your shoulders relaxed.

2. Place your palms on your forehead, with your fingers spread out and facing upward.

3. Gently smooth your palms over your forehead, moving from the center of your forehead outward toward your temples.

4. As you smooth your palms outward, use your fingertips to apply gentle pressure to the skin, which can help to stimulate blood flow and promote relaxation.

5. Repeat this exercise several times, taking deep breaths in between each repetition.

The Forehead Wrinkle Smoother pose targets the muscles in the forehead, including the frontalis muscle, which is responsible for raising the eyebrows and creating wrinkles on the forehead. By performing this exercise regularly, you can help to tone and strengthen these muscles, which can reduce the appearance of wrinkles and fine lines in the forehead area. Additionally, this pose can help to relieve tension in the forehead and promote relaxation in the face and mind.

The Eyebrow Furrow Smoother

The Eyebrow Furrow Smoother is a facial exercise that is designed to help improve the appearance of the forehead and surrounding area. It works by exercising the muscles of the forehead, which can help to smooth and reduce the appearance of fine lines and wrinkles in this area. This exercise can be used to address a variety of face appearance issues, including:

- *Fine lines and wrinkles in the forehead and surrounding area*

- *Sagging skin in the forehead and surrounding area*

- *Poor posture, which can contribute to the appearance of fine lines and wrinkles*

It is a non-invasive way to improve the appearance of the forehead and surrounding area and overall facial appearance.

The Eyebrow Furrow Smoother can help tone and relax the muscles around the eyes and forehead. This pose primarily targets **the corrugator muscles**, which are located between the eyebrows and are responsible for creating vertical lines or furrows on the forehead.

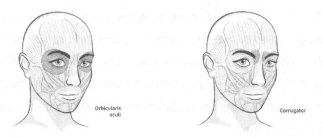

To perform The Eyebrow Furrow Smoother, you place your index fingers above each eyebrow and press gently while moving the skin around the eyebrows up and down. This helps to relax and tone the corrugator muscles, reducing the appearance of wrinkles and furrows between the eyebrows.

In addition to the corrugator muscles, this pose may also engage other muscles in the face, including **the orbicularis oculi muscles**, which are responsible for closing the eyes tightly. By engaging these muscles and promoting relaxation, The Eyebrow Furrow Smoother can help improve overall facial muscle tone and promote a more youthful appearance around the eyes and forehead.

The technique involves placing the index fingers above each

eyebrow and pressing gently while moving the skin around the eyebrows up and down. This helps to relax and tone the corrugator muscles, reducing the appearance of wrinkles and furrows between the eyebrows. This pose can be a helpful addition to a regular facial yoga practice for those looking to tone and rejuvenate the muscles of the face.

Here's how to do it:

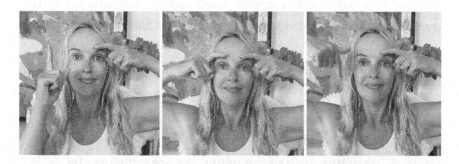

Apply some facial oil to the palms of your hands and then massage it onto your face and neck, making sure to cover all areas where you will be performing Face Yoga exercises.

1. Sit or stand in a comfortable position with your back straight and your shoulders relaxed.

2. Place your index fingers above each eyebrow, with the tips of your fingers pointing towards each other.

3. Apply gentle pressure with your fingers, and start moving the skin around

4. your eyebrows up and down. You should feel the muscles between your eyebrows engaging.

5. Continue to move the skin up and down for about 30 seconds, breathing deeply and relaxing your facial muscles.

6. Release your fingers, and take a few deep breaths to relax your facial muscles.

7. Repeat the exercise for 2-3 sets, with a short break in between each set.

The Eyebrow Furrow Smoother can help tone and relax the corrugator muscles, reducing the appearance of wrinkles and furrows between the eyebrows. With regular practice, this exercise can help improve overall facial muscle tone and promote a more youthful appearance around the eyes and forehead.

The Eye Bag Reducer

The Eye Bag Reducer is a facial exercise that is designed to help improve the appearance of the under-eye area. It works by exercising the muscles of the under-eye area, which can help to tighten and tone the skin in this area. This exercise can be used to address a variety of face appearance issues, including:

- *Dark circles and puffiness under the eyes*

- *Sagging skin in the under-eye area*

- *Fine lines and wrinkles in the under-eye area*

- *Poor circulation, which can contribute to the appearance of dark circles and puffiness under the eyes*

The Eye Bag Reducer can help tone and rejuvenate the muscles around the eyes and reduce the appearance of under-eye bags or puffiness.

The Eye Bag Reducer primarily targets **the orbicularis oculi muscle.** The orbicularis oculi muscle is a facial muscle that encircles the eye and is responsible for eyelid closure and blinking. It is divided into two parts: the palpebral part, which is responsible for eyelid closure, and the orbital part, which is responsible for wrinkles around the eyes, such as crow's feet. When performing the Eye Bag Reducer, the gentle pressure on the outer and inner corners of the eyes can help tone and strengthen both parts of the orbicularis oculi muscle, resulting in a more toned and youthful appearance around the eyes.

To perform The Eye Bag Reducer, you place your index and middle fingers on the inner corners of your eyebrows and your ring and little fingers on the outer corners of your eyes. You then apply gentle pressure with your fingers and look up towards the ceiling, as if trying to lift your eyelids.

Here's how to do it:

Apply some facial oil to the palms of your hands and then massage it onto your face and neck, making sure to cover all areas where you will be performing Face Yoga exercises.

1. Sit or stand in a comfortable position with your back straight and your shoulders relaxed.

2. Place your index and middle fingers on the inner corners of your eyebrows, and your ring and little fingers on the outer corners of your eyes.

3. Apply gentle pressure with your fingers and look up towards the ceiling, as if trying to lift your eyelids.

4. Hold the pose for 10-15 seconds, breathing deeply and relaxing your facial muscles.

5. Release the pose and take a few deep breaths to relax your facial muscles.

6. Repeat the exercise for 2-3 sets, with a short break in between each set.

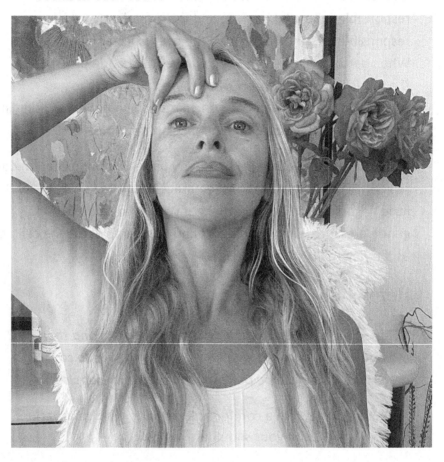

By holding this pose, you can tone and strengthen **the orbicularis oculi muscles,** which can help reduce the appearance of under-eye bags or puffiness. The gentle pressure from your fingers can also help promote lymphatic drainage and reduce swelling in the eye area.

Overall, The Eye Bag Reducer can help improve the muscle tone and circulation around the eyes, resulting in a more youthful and refreshed appearance. It can be a helpful addition to a regular facial yoga practice for those looking to reduce under-eye bags *and puffiness.*

With regular practice, this pose can also help improve overall facial muscle tone and promote a more youthful appearance around the eyes.

The Lip Pout

The Lip Pout is a facial exercise that is designed to help improve the appearance of the lips and surrounding area. It works by exercising the muscles of the lips and cheek, which can help to tighten and tone the skin in this area. This exercise can be used to address a variety of face appearance issues, including:

- *Sagging skin around the mouth*

- *Fine lines and wrinkles around the mouth and cheek area*

- *Poor posture, which can contribute to the appearance of fine lines and wrinkles*

The Lip Pout can help tone and firm the muscles around the mouth, promoting a fuller, more youthful appearance.

This pose that primarily targets the **orbicularis oris muscle**. This muscle encircles the mouth and is responsible for puckering the lips and producing facial expressions related to speech and kissing. The orbicularis oris muscle also plays an important role in maintaining the shape and fullness of the lips.

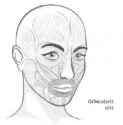
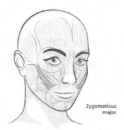
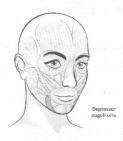

Orbicularis oris

Zygomaticus major

Depressor auguli oris

When performing The Lip Pout, you extend your lips as far out as possible, engaging and toning the orbicularis oris muscle. This can help firm and tone the muscles around the mouth, promoting a fuller and more youthful appearance.

The Lip Pout may also engage other muscles in the face, such as the **zygomaticus major muscle**, which is responsible for smiling, and the **depressor anguli oris** muscle, which is responsible for frowning. By engaging and toning these muscles, The Lip Pout can help improve overall facial muscle tone and promote a more youthful appearance.

Overall, The Lip Pout is a beneficial facial yoga pose for those looking to tone and firm the muscles around the mouth, promoting a fuller and more youthful appearance.

Here's how to do it:

Apply some facial oil to the palms of your hands and then massage it onto your face and neck, making sure to cover all areas where you will be performing Face Yoga exercises.

1. Sit or stand in a comfortable position with your back straight and your shoulders relaxed.

2. Pout your lips as if you are about to kiss someone, extending your lips as far out as possible.

3. Hold the pose for 5-10 seconds, breathing deeply and relaxing your facial muscles.

4. Release the pose and take a few deep breaths to relax your facial muscles.

5. Repeat the exercise for 2-3 sets, with a short break in between each set.

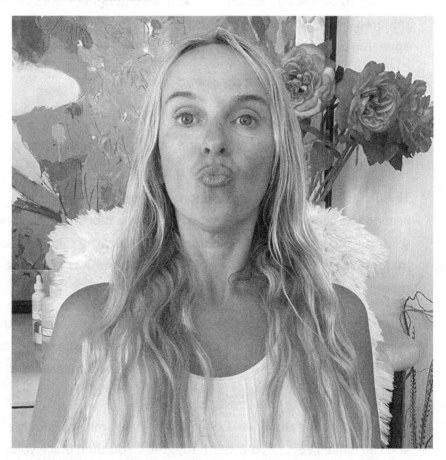

The Lip Pout can help tone and firm the orbicularis oris muscle, promoting a fuller and more youthful appearance around the mouth. With regular practice, this pose can also help improve overall facial muscle tone and promote a more youthful appearance.

The Cheekbone Definer

The Cheekbone Definer is a facial exercise that is designed to help improve the appearance of the cheekbones and surrounding area. It works by exercising the muscles of the cheek and jaw, which can help to define and lift the cheekbones and tighten the skin in this area. This exercise can be used to address a variety of face appearance issues, including:

- *Sagging skin in the cheek and jaw area*

- *A weak or undefined jawline*

- *Poor posture, which can contribute to the appearance of sagging skin*

The Cheekbone Definer can help tone and define the muscles around the cheeks and cheekbones, creating a more sculpted and youthful appearance. This pose primarily targets the **zygomaticus major muscle**, which is responsible for raising the corners of the mouth and creating the appearance of smiling.

The zygomaticus major muscle is a facial muscle that connects the zygomatic bone to the corner of the mouth and is responsible for raising the corners of the mouth and creating the appearance of smiling.

When performing the Cheekbone Definer, you smile as widely as you can while keeping your teeth together. You then place your index fingers on the top of your cheekbones and press gently upwards towards your eyes. By doing this, you engage and tone the zygomaticus major muscle, promoting a more sculpted and youthful appearance around the cheeks and cheekbones.

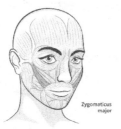 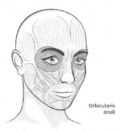

In addition to the zygomaticus major muscle, The Cheekbone Definer may also engage other muscles in the face, such as the **orbicularis oculi muscle**, which is responsible for closing the eyes tightly. By engaging and toning these muscles, this pose can help improve overall facial muscle tone and promote a more youthful appearance.

Overall, The Cheekbone Definer is a beneficial facial yoga pose for those looking to tone and define the muscles around the cheeks and cheekbones, creating a more sculpted and youthful appearance.

Here's how to do it:

Apply some facial oil to the palms of your hands and then massage it onto your face and neck, making sure to cover all areas where you will be performing Face Yoga exercises.

1. Sit or stand in a comfortable position with your back straight and your shoulders relaxed.

2. Smile as widely as you can, making sure to keep your teeth together.

3. Place your index fingers on the top of your cheekbones, and press gently upwards towards your eyes.

4. Hold the pose for 10-15 seconds, breathing deeply and relaxing your facial muscles.

5. Release the pose and take a few deep breaths to relax your facial muscles.

6. Repeat the exercise for 2-3 sets, with a short break in between each set.

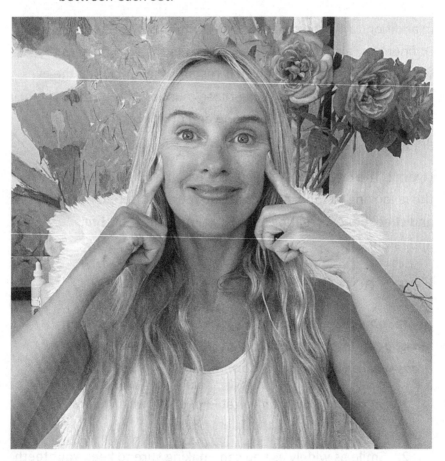

The Cheekbone Definer can help tone and define the zygomaticus major muscle, promoting a more sculpted and youthful appearance around the cheeks and cheekbones. With regular practice, this pose can also help improve overall facial muscle tone and promote a more youthful appearance.

The Double Chin Reducer

The Double Chin Reducer is a facial exercise that is designed to help improve the appearance of the neck and chin area. It works by exercising the muscles of the neck and chin, which can help to tighten and tone the skin in this area. This exercise can be used to address a variety of face appearance issues, including:

- *A double chin*

- *Sagging skin in the neck and chin area*

- *Poor posture, which can contribute to the appearance of a double chin*

The Double Chin Reducer can help tone and strengthen the muscles around the chin and neck, reducing the appearance of a double chin. This pose primarily targets **the platysma muscle,** which is a thin sheet of muscle that extends from the collarbone to the jawline and is responsible for moving the jaw and lower lip.

When the platysma muscle is weak or loose, it can contribute to the appearance of a double chin.

The Double Chin Reducer pose involves tilting the head back and looking up towards the ceiling, while pressing the tongue against the roof of the mouth and sliding it backwards towards the back of the mouth. This engages and tones the muscles around the chin and neck, particularly the platysma muscle. With regular practice, this pose can help strengthen and tone the platysma muscle, reducing the appearance of a double chin and promoting a more defined and toned appearance around the chin and neck.

In addition to the platysma muscle, The Double Chin Reducer may also engage other muscles in the face and neck, such as the muscles in the jawline and upper neck. By engaging and toning these muscles, this pose can help improve overall facial muscle tone and promote a more youthful appearance.

Here's how to do it:

Apply some facial oil to the palms of your hands and then massage it onto your face and neck, making sure to cover all areas where you will be performing Face Yoga exercises.

1. Sit or stand in a comfortable position with your back straight and your shoulders relaxed.

2. Tilt your head back and look up towards the ceiling.

3. Press your tongue against the roof of your mouth, and slide it backwards towards the back of your mouth.

4. Hold the pose for 5-10 seconds, breathing deeply and relaxing your facial muscles.

5. Release the pose and take a few deep breaths to relax your facial muscles.

6. Repeat the exercise for 2-3 sets, with a short break in between each set.

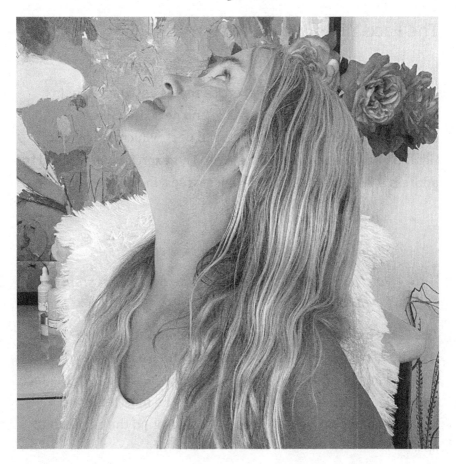

The Double Chin Reducer can help tone and strengthen the platysma muscle, reducing the appearance of a double chin. The pressing of the tongue against the roof of the mouth and the sliding of the tongue backwards can help engage and tone the muscles around the chin and neck, resulting in a more defined and toned appearance. With regular practice, this pose can also help improve overall facial muscle tone and promote a more youthful appearance.

The Face Slimming Exercise

The Face Slimming is a facial exercise that is designed to help improve the appearance of the face and neck. It works by exercising the muscles of the face and neck, which can help to tighten and tone the skin in this area. This exercise can be used to address a variety of face appearance issues, including:

- *A full or rounded face*

- *Sagging skin in the face and neck area*

- *Poor posture, which can contribute to the appearance of a full or rounded face*

The Face Slimming Exercise can help tone and strengthen the muscles around the face and neck, promoting a more defined and sculpted appearance. This pose targets several muscles in the face and neck, including the platysma muscle, the muscles in the jawline and upper neck, and the muscles around the cheeks and lips.

This exercise targets several muscles in the face and neck, including **the platysma muscle**, the muscles in the jawline and upper neck, and the muscles around the cheeks and lips.

The Face Slimming Exercise engages and tones several muscles in the face and neck, including:

1. **The platysma muscle** - A thin sheet of muscle that extends from the collarbone to the jawline and is responsible for moving the jaw and lower lip. This muscle is engaged when making the "O" shape with the mouth, helping to tone and reduce the appearance of a double chin.

2. **The muscles in the jawline and upper neck** - These muscles play an important role in defining and sculpting the appearance of the face. Engaging and toning these muscles can promote a more toned and youthful look.

3. **The muscles around the cheeks and lips** - These muscles are engaged by making the "O" shape with the mouth, promoting a more defined and sculpted appearance around the cheeks and lips.

The platysma muscle extends from the collarbone to the jawline and is responsible for moving the jaw and lower lip. When the platysma muscle is weak or loose, it can contribute to the appearance of a double chin. The "O" shape of the mouth in this pose can help engage and tone the platysma muscle, reducing the appearance of a double chin.

The muscles in the jawline and upper neck are also engaged in this pose. These muscles play an important role in defining and sculpting the appearance of the face and can contribute to the appearance of a more toned and youthful look.

The muscles around the cheeks and lips are also engaged in this pose. By making the "O" shape with the mouth, you engage and tone these muscles, promoting a more defined and sculpted appearance around the cheeks and lips.

Overall, The Face Slimming Exercise is a beneficial facial yoga pose for those looking to tone and strengthen the muscles around the face and neck, promoting a more defined and sculpted appearance.

Here's how to do it:

Apply some facial oil to the palms of your hands and then

massage it onto your face and neck, making sure to cover all areas where you will be performing Face Yoga exercises.

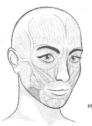 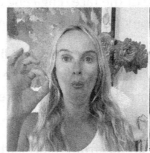 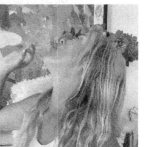

Platysma

1. Sit or stand in a comfortable position with your back straight and your shoulders relaxed.

2. Tilt your head back and look up towards the ceiling.

3. Close your lips and make an "O" shape with your mouth.

4. Hold the pose for 5-10 seconds, breathing deeply and relaxing your facial muscles.

5. Release the pose and take a few deep breaths to relax your facial muscles.

6. Repeat the exercise for 2-3 sets, with a short break in between each set.

By performing this pose, you engage and tone the muscles around the face and neck, particularly the platysma muscle, which can help reduce the appearance of a double chin. The "O" shape of the mouth can also help tone and strengthen the muscles around the cheeks and lips, promoting a more defined and sculpted appearance.

With regular practice, this pose can help improve overall facial muscle tone and promote a more youthful appearance.

Overall, The Face Slimming Exercise is a beneficial facial yoga pose for those looking to tone and strengthen the muscles around the face and neck, promoting a more defined and sculpted appearance.

The Nose Scrunch

The Nose Scrunch is a facial exercise that is designed to help improve the appearance of the nose and surrounding area. It works by exercising the muscles of the nose and surrounding area, which can help to tighten and tone the skin in this area. This exercise can be used to address a variety of face appearance issues, including:

- *A flat or undefined nose*

- *Poor posture, which can contribute to the appearance of a flat or undefined nose*

- *Fine lines and wrinkles in the nose and surrounding area*

- *Sagging skin in the nose and surrounding area*

The Nose Scrunch is a non-invasive way to improve the appearance of the nose and surrounding area and overall facial appearance.

This exercise can help tone and strengthen the muscles around the nose and mouth, promoting a more youthful and defined appearance. This pose primarily targets the nasalis muscle, which is a facial muscle that runs along the sides of the nose and is responsible for flaring and scrunching the nostrils. This muscle plays an important role in facial expressions related to smelling, such as wrinkling the nose in response to an unpleasant odor.

When performing The Nose Scrunch, you wrinkle your nose and flare your nostrils as much as possible. This engages and tones **the nasalis muscle**, promoting a more youthful and defined appearance around the nose and mouth. With regular practice, this pose can also help improve overall facial muscle tone and promote a more youthful appearance.

In addition to the nasalis muscle, The Nose Scrunch may also engage other muscles in the face, such as **the procerus muscle** and the **levator labii superioris alaeque nasi muscle**. These muscles are involved in wrinkling the skin around the nose and upper lip, and can also be toned and strengthened through regular practice of this pose.

The Nose Scrunch Exercise engages and tones several muscles in the face, including:

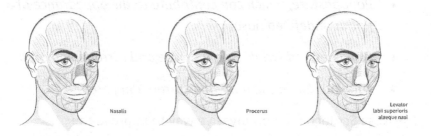

1. **The nasalis muscle** - This muscle runs along the sides of the nose and is responsible for flaring and scrunching the nostrils. The Nasalis muscle is the primary muscle engaged in this pose.

2. **The procerus muscle** - This muscle is located between the eyebrows and is responsible for wrinkling the skin in that area.

3. **The levator labii superioris alaeque nasi muscle** - This muscle is located between the upper lip and the nose and is responsible for lifting the upper lip and flaring the nostrils.

Here's how to do it:

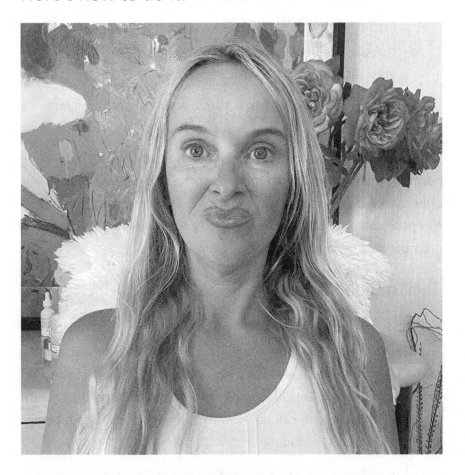

Apply some facial oil to the palms of your hands and then massage it onto your face and neck, making sure to cover all areas where you will be performing Face Yoga exercises.

1. Sit or stand in a comfortable position with your back straight and your shoulders relaxed.

2. Wrinkle your nose and flare your nostrils as much as possible.

3. Hold the pose for 5-10 seconds, breathing deeply and relaxing your facial muscles.

4. Release the pose and take a few deep breaths to relax your facial muscles.

5. Repeat the exercise for 2-3 sets, with a short break in between each set.

The Nose Scrunch Exercise can help tone and strengthen the nasalis muscle, promoting a more youthful and defined appearance around the nose and mouth. With regular practice, this pose can also help improve overall facial muscle tone and promote a more youthful appearance.

The Tongue Stretch

The Tongue Stretch is designed to help improve the appearance of the face and neck. It works by exercising the muscles of the face, neck, and jaw, which can help to tighten and tone the skin in this area. This exercise can be used to address a variety of face appearance issues, including:

- *Sagging skin in the face and neck area*

- *Poor posture, which can contribute to the appearance of sagging skin*

- *Fine lines and wrinkles in the face and neck area*

- *A weak or undefined jawline*

The Tongue Stretch can help tone and strengthen the muscles around the face and neck, promoting a more defined and youthful appearance. This pose primarily targets the muscles in the tongue and the muscles in the neck.

By sticking out your tongue as far as possible and pointing it downwards towards your chin, you engage and tone the muscles in the tongue. These muscles play an important role in speech and swallowing and can also contribute to the appearance of a more toned and youthful look around the mouth.

In addition to the **muscles in the tongue,** The Tongue Stretch also engages and tones the **muscles in the neck**. By stretching the tongue downwards towards the chin, you engage and tone the muscles in the neck, which can help reduce sagging and promote a more defined appearance.

Overall, The Tongue Stretch is a beneficial facial yoga pose for those looking to tone and strengthen the muscles around the tongue and neck, promoting a more defined and youthful appearance.

Here's how to do it:

Apply some facial oil to the palms of your hands and then massage it onto your face and neck, making sure to cover all areas where you will be performing Face Yoga exercises.

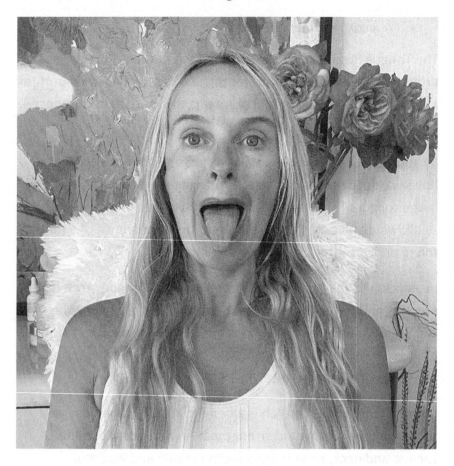

1. Sit or stand in a comfortable position with your back straight and your shoulders relaxed.

2. Stick out your tongue as far as possible and point it downwards towards your chin.

3. Hold the pose for 5-10 seconds, breathing deeply and relaxing your facial muscles.

4. Bring your tongue back into your mouth and relax your tongue and facial muscles.

5. Repeat the exercise for 2-3 sets, with a short break in between each set.

It is a non-invasive way to improve the appearance of the mouth and surrounding area and overall facial appearance.

The Mouth Corner Lift can help tone and strengthen the muscles around the mouth, promoting a more defined and youthful appearance. This pose primarily targets the zygomaticus major and minor muscles, which are muscles that run from the cheekbone to the corners of the mouth and are responsible for lifting the corners of the mouth.

This pose primarily targets the **zygomaticus major and minor muscles.**

By lifting the corners of the mouth upwards towards the fingers, you engage and tone the zygomaticus major and minor muscles. This can help reduce the appearance of fine lines and wrinkles around the mouth, as well as promote a more defined and youthful appearance around the mouth.

In addition to the zygomaticus major and minor muscles, the Mouth Corner Lift may also engage other muscles in the face, such as **the orbicularis oris muscle** and **the levator anguli oris muscle**. These muscles are involved in shaping the lips and can also be toned and strengthened through regular practice of this pose.

1. **The zygomaticus major and minor muscles** - These muscles run from the cheekbone to the corners of the mouth and are responsible for lifting the corners of the mouth.
2. **The orbicularis oris muscle** - This muscle is located around the lips and is responsible for shaping the lips during facial expressions such as smiling, pouting, and whistling.

3. **The levator anguli oris muscle** - This muscle is located at the corner of the mouth and is responsible for lifting the corner of the mouth upwards, similar to the zygomaticus muscles.

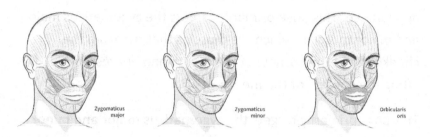

Zygomaticus major   Zygomaticus minor   Orbicularis oris

Overall, the Mouth Corner Lift can help tone and strengthen the zygomaticus major and minor muscles, as well as other muscles involved in shaping the lips, promoting a more defined and youthful appearance around the mouth.

Here's how to do it:

Apply some facial oil to the palms of your hands and then massage it onto your face and neck, making sure to cover all areas where you will be performing Face Yoga exercises.

1. Sit or stand in a comfortable position with your back straight and your shoulders relaxed.

2. Place your index fingers at the corners of your mouth, with your fingers pointing upwards.

3. Gently lift the corners of your mouth upwards towards your fingers, while keeping your lips closed.

4. Hold the pose for 5-10 seconds, breathing deeply and relaxing your facial muscles.

5. Release the pose and take a few deep breaths to relax your facial muscles.

6. Repeat the exercise for 2-3 sets, with a short break in between each set.

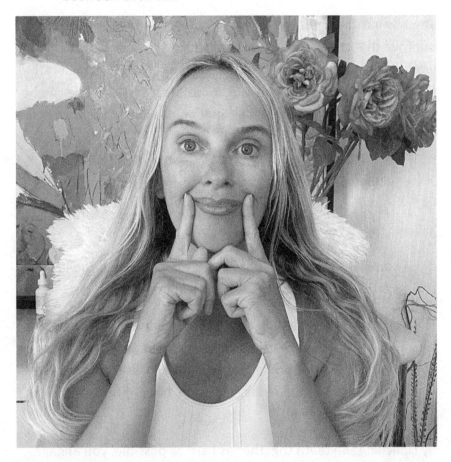

The Mouth Corner Lift Exercise can help tone and strengthen the zygomaticus major and minor muscles, promoting a more defined and youthful appearance around the mouth. By lifting the corners of the mouth upwards towards the fingers, you engage and tone these muscles, which can help reduce the appearance of fine lines and wrinkles around the mouth. With regular practice, this pose can also help improve overall facial muscle tone and promote a

more youthful appearance.

The Jawline Toner

The Jawline Toner Lift is a facial exercise that is designed to help improve the appearance of the jawline and surrounding area. It works by exercising the muscles of the jaw and neck, which can help to tighten and tone the skin in this area. This exercise can be used to address a variety of face appearance issues, including:

- *A weak or undefined jawline*

- *Sagging skin in the jaw and neck area*

- *Poor posture, which can contribute to the appearance of a weak or undefined jawline*

It is a non-invasive way to improve the appearance of the jawline and surrounding area and overall facial appearance.

This yoga pose that can help tone and strengthen the muscles around the jawline, promoting a more defined and youthful appearance. This pose primarily targets **the masseter muscle**, which is a powerful muscle located at the back of the jaw and is responsible for chewing.

By clenching the teeth together as hard as possible, you engage and tone the masseter muscle. This can help reduce the appearance of sagging around the jawline and promote a more defined and youthful appearance.

In addition to the masseter muscle, the Jawline Toner Exercise may also engage other muscles in the face, including:

These muscles are involved in chewing and neck movements and can also be toned and strengthened through regular practice of this pose. Overall, the Jawline Toner Exercise is a beneficial facial yoga pose for those looking to tone and strengthen the muscles around the jawline, promoting a more defined and youthful appearance.

Here's how to do it:

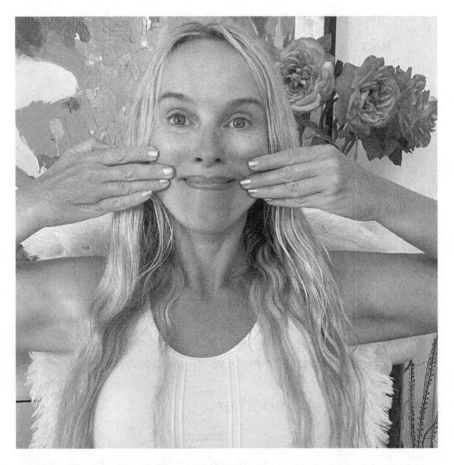

Apply some facial oil to the palms of your hands and then massage it onto your face and neck, making sure to cover all areas where you will be performing Face Yoga exercises.

1. Sit or stand in a comfortable position with your back straight and your shoulders relaxed.

2. Place your fingers on the sides of your face, just below your cheekbones.

3. Clench your teeth together as hard as possible, while keeping your lips closed.

4. Feel the muscle bulging on the sides of your face.

5. Hold the pose for 5-10 seconds, breathing deeply and relaxing your facial muscles.

6. Release the pose and take a few deep breaths to relax your facial muscles.

7. Repeat the exercise for 2-3 sets, with a short break in between each set.

The Jawline Toner Exercise can help tone and strengthen the masseter muscle, promoting a more defined and youthful appearance around the jawline. By clenching your teeth together as hard as possible, you engage and tone the masseter muscle, which can help reduce the appearance of sagging and promote a more defined and youthful appearance around the jawline. With regular practice, this pose can also help improve overall facial muscle tone and promote a more youthful appearance.

The Crow's Feet Smoother

The Crow's Feet Smoother is a facial exercise that is designed to help improve the appearance of the eye area, including the crow's feet. It works by exercising the muscles of the eye and surrounding area, which can help to tighten and tone the skin in this area. This exercise can be used to address a variety of face appearance issues, including:

- *Fine lines and wrinkles around the eyes, including crow's feet*

- *Sagging skin in the eye and surrounding area*

- *Poor posture, which can contribute to the appearance of fine lines and wrinkles around the eyes*

It can help tone and strengthen the muscles around the eyes, promoting a more youthful and rested appearance. This pose primarily targets the orbicularis oculi muscle, which is a circular muscle that surrounds the eye and is responsible for closing the eyelids.

By closing the eyes tightly while pulling the skin outwards and upwards towards the temples, you engage and tone the orbicularis oculi muscle. This can help reduce the appearance of fine lines and wrinkles around the eyes, promoting a more youthful and rested appearance.

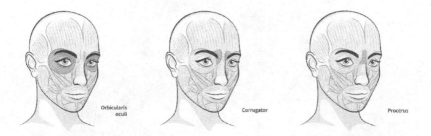

In addition to **the orbicularis oculi muscle**, The Crow's Feet Smoother Exercise may also engage other muscles in the face, such as **the corrugator supercilii** muscle and **the procerus muscle.** These muscles are involved in facial expressions of worry, concern, or anger, and can also be toned and strengthened through regular practice of this pose.

In summary, The Crow's Feet Smoother Exercise can be a useful facial yoga pose for anyone seeking to tone and strengthen the muscles around the eyes. This pose can help reduce the appearance of fine lines and wrinkles around the eyes, resulting in a more youthful and rested appearance.

Here's how to do it:

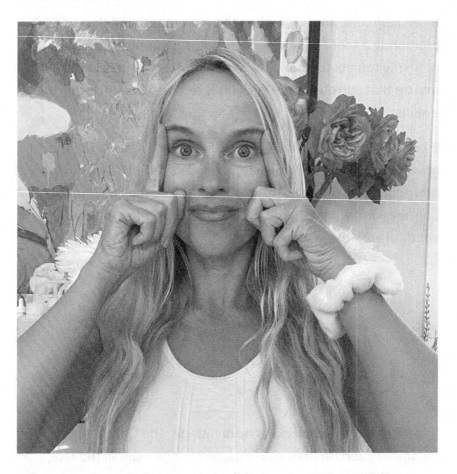

Apply some facial oil to the palms of your hands and then massage it onto your face and neck, making sure to cover all

areas where you will be performing Face Yoga exercises.

1. Sit or stand in a comfortable position with your back straight and your shoulders relaxed.

2. Place your index fingers at the outer corners of your eyes, with your fingers pointing towards your temples.

3. Gently pull your skin outwards and upwards towards your temples.

4. Close your eyes as tightly as possible, while keeping your fingers in place.

5. Hold the pose for 5-10 seconds, breathing deeply and relaxing your facial muscles.

6. Release the pose and take a few deep breaths to relax your facial muscles.

7. Repeat the exercise for 2-3 sets, with a short break in between each set.

The Crow's Feet Smoother Exercise can help tone and strengthen the orbicularis oculi muscle, promoting a more youthful and rested appearance around the eyes. By pulling the skin outwards and upwards while closing the eyes tightly, you engage and tone the orbicularis oculi muscle, which can help reduce the appearance of fine lines and wrinkles around the eyes. With regular practice, this pose can also help improve overall facial muscle tone and promote a more youthful appearance.

The Forehead Press

The Forehead Press is a facial exercise that is designed to help improve the appearance of the forehead and surrounding area. It works by exercising the muscles of the forehead, which can help to tighten and tone the skin in this area. This exercise can be used to address a variety of face appearance issues, including:

- *Fine lines and wrinkles in the forehead and surrounding area*

- *Sagging skin in the forehead and surrounding area*

- *Poor posture, which can contribute to the appearance of fine lines and wrinkles*

It is a non-invasive way to improve the appearance of the forehead and surrounding area and overall facial appearance. This exercise that can help to tone and firm the muscles in the forehead and around the eyes.

There are numerous muscles in the face, some of which are involved in facial expressions and others that are involved in other functions such as chewing and speaking.

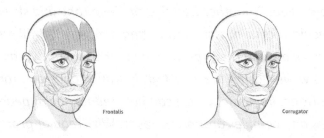

The Forehead Press exercise in Face Yoga mainly targets **the frontalis muscle,** which is the muscle located at the front of the forehead. This muscle is responsible for raising the eyebrows and creating horizontal wrinkles on the forehead.

Additionally, The Forehead Press exercise can also engage **the corrugator muscles,** which are the small muscles located between the eyebrows. These muscles are responsible for creating vertical wrinkles between the eyebrows and can also contribute to tension in the forehead area.

By practicing The Forehead Press exercise regularly, these muscles can be toned and strengthened, which may help to improve the overall appearance of the forehead and eye area.

Here's how to do it:

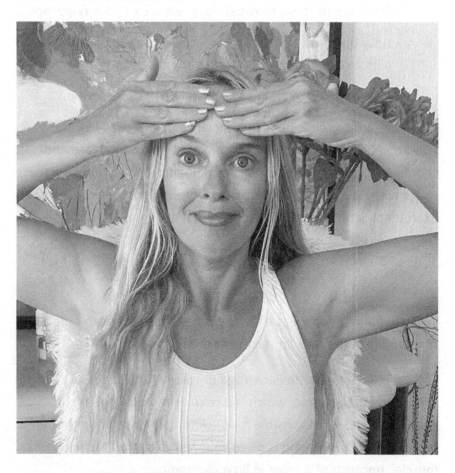

Apply some facial oil to the palms of your hands and then massage it onto your face and neck, making sure to cover all

areas where you will be performing Face Yoga exercises.

1. Start by sitting comfortably with your back straight and your shoulders relaxed.

2. Place your fingertips on your forehead, just above your eyebrows.

3. Gently press your fingertips into your skin and slide them upwards, towards your hairline. As you do this, use your forehead muscles to resist the pressure of your fingertips.

4. Hold this position for a few seconds, then release the pressure and allow your forehead muscles to relax.

5. Repeat this movement for a total of 10-15 repetitions.

It's important to remember that facial yoga exercises like The Forehead Press should be performed gently and with care and should not cause any discomfort or pain. It's also a good idea to check with your healthcare provider before beginning any new exercise program, including facial yoga.

The Lip Balm

The "Lip Balm" exercise is a facial yoga exercise that can help to tone and firm the muscles around the mouth and lips.

The Lip Balm exercise in Face Yoga primarily targets **the orbicularis oris muscle**, which is a circular muscle that encircles the mouth and is responsible for puckering the lips and other lip movements. This muscle is often referred to as the "kissing muscle" because of its role in lip movements.

Additionally, The Lip Balm exercise can also engage other muscles around the mouth and lips, including **the depressor labii muscles** and **the mentalis muscle.** The depressor labii muscles are located on either side of the chin and are responsible for pulling the lower lip downwards, while the mentalis muscle is located on the chin and is responsible for chin movements.

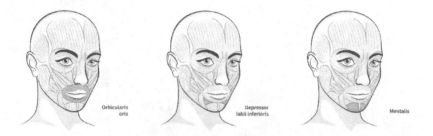

1. **Orbicularis oris muscle**: a circular muscle that encircles the mouth and is responsible for puckering the lips and other lip movements.

2. **Depressor labii muscles:** a pair of muscles located on either side of the chin and are responsible for pulling the lower lip downwards.

3. **Mentalis muscle:** a muscle located on the chin and is responsible for chin movements.

By practicing The Lip Balm exercise regularly, these muscles can be toned and strengthened, which may help to improve the overall appearance of the mouth and lip area.

Here's how to do it:

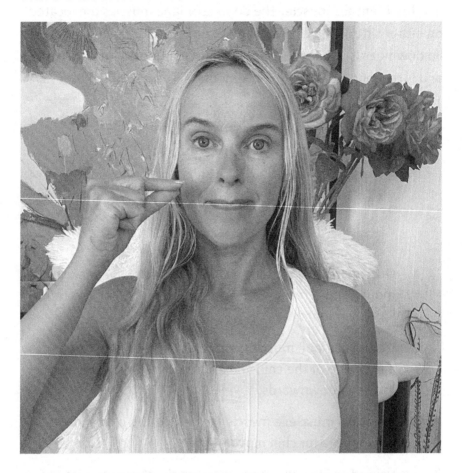

Apply some facial oil to the palms of your hands and then massage it onto your face and neck, making sure to cover all areas where you will be performing Face Yoga exercises.

1. Start by sitting comfortably with your back straight and your shoulders relaxed.

2. Close your mouth and press your lips together firmly.

3. Hold this position for a few seconds, then release the pressure and allow your lips to relax.

4. Next, pucker your lips outwards, as if you were applying lip balm to your lips.

5. Hold this position for a few seconds, then release the pressure and allow your lips to relax.

6. Repeat these two movements (pressing the lips together and puckering the lips) for a total of 10-15 repetitions.

It's important to remember to perform this exercise gently and with care to avoid any discomfort or strain. It's also a good idea to check with your healthcare provider before beginning any new exercise program, including facial yoga.

The Tongue Twister

The Tongue Twister is a facial yoga exercise that can help to tone and firm the muscles in the face, especially those around the mouth, tongue, and cheeks.

These muscles include:

1. **Orbicularis oris muscle:** a circular muscle that encircles the mouth and is responsible for puckering the lips and other lip movements.

2. **Buccinator muscles:** a pair of muscles located in the cheeks that help to pull the cheeks inwards and assist with movements like chewing and speaking.

3. **Tongue muscles:** a group of muscles in the tongue that are responsible for moving the tongue in different directions and shapes.

By practicing The Tongue Twister exercise regularly, these muscles can be toned and strengthened, which may help to improve the overall appearance and tone of the face. Additionally, this exercise can help to improve speech and enunciation by strengthening the tongue muscles. It's important to note that facial yoga exercises should be performed gently and with care to avoid any discomfort or strain.

Here's how to do it:

Apply some facial oil to the palms of your hands and then massage it onto your face and neck, making sure to cover all areas where you will be performing Face Yoga exercises.

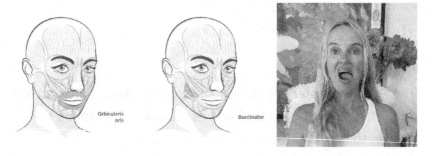

1. Start by sitting comfortably with your back straight and your shoulders relaxed.

2. Open your mouth wide and stick out your tongue as far as you can.

3. Move your tongue around in a circular motion, touching the outer edges of your upper and lower teeth as you do so.

4. Next, say the following tongue twister while continuing to move your tongue around: "red lorry, yellow lorry" (or any other tongue twister of your choice).

5. Repeat this movement and tongue twister for a total of 10-15 repetitions.

It's important to perform this exercise gently and with care to avoid any discomfort or strain. It's also a good idea to check with your healthcare provider before beginning any new exercise program, including facial yoga.

The Nose Massage

The Nose Massage is a simple, yet effective Face Yoga pose that can help to relieve tension and improve blood circulation in the facial muscles.

It is designed to help improve the appearance of the nose and surrounding area. It works by massaging the muscles and skin of the nose and surrounding area, which can help to improve circulation and promote lymphatic drainage. This exercise can be used to address a variety of face appearance issues, including:

- *Puffy or swollen appearance in the nose and surrounding area*

- *Fine lines and wrinkles in the nose and surrounding area*

- *Poor circulation, which can contribute to puffiness or a dull appearance in the skin*

The Nose Massage exercise in Face Yoga primarily targets the muscles in the nose area, including **the nasalis muscle** and **the procerus muscle.** These muscles are responsible for the movement of the nostrils and the skin around the nose, respectively.

The nasalis muscle is a paired muscle that runs from the bridge of the nose down to the nostrils. This muscle is responsible for flaring the nostrils and compressing the nasal cartilages.

The procerus muscle is a small, triangular muscle located between the eyebrows. This muscle is responsible for pulling the skin between the eyebrows downward, creating vertical wrinkles known as frown lines.

During The Nose Massage exercise, the gentle circular motion applied to the bridge and sides of the nose helps to improve blood flow to the muscles in this area. This increased blood flow can help to relieve tension and promote relaxation in the muscles, reducing the appearance of fine lines and wrinkles and improving overall facial tone.

Additionally, The Nose Massage exercise can also help to stimulate the flow of oxygen and nutrients to the facial muscles, which can improve the health and appearance of the skin. By performing this exercise regularly, you can help to maintain healthy facial muscles and reduce the signs of aging in the nose area.

Here's how to do it:

Apply some facial oil to the palms of your hands and then massage it onto your face and neck, making sure to cover all areas where you will be performing Face Yoga exercises.

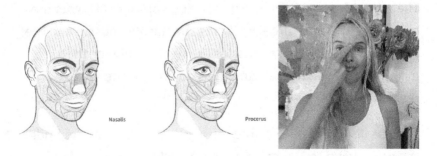

Nasalis   Procerus

1. Sit in a comfortable position with your back straight and your shoulders relaxed.

2. Place your index and middle fingers on the bridge of your nose, just below the eyebrows.

3. Apply gentle pressure with your fingers and massage the area in a circular motion for 30 seconds.

4. Move your fingers down to the sides of your nose and repeat the circular massage motion for another 30 seconds.

5. Finally, place your fingers on the sides of your nostrils and massage in a circular motion for 30 seconds.

6. Repeat the entire sequence 2-3 times.

The Nose Massage exercise can help to stimulate the flow of oxygen and nutrients to the facial muscles, which can improve skin tone and reduce the appearance of fine lines and wrinkles. Additionally, this exercise can help to relieve tension in the sinus area, which can be beneficial for people who suffer from allergies or sinus congestion.

The Temple Toner

The Temple Toner Facial Yoga Pose is a facial exercise that is designed to help improve the appearance of the temple and surrounding area. It works by exercising the muscles of the temple and surrounding area, which can help to tighten and tone the skin in this area. This exercise can be used to address a variety of face appearance issues, including:

- *Fine lines and wrinkles in the temple and surrounding area*

- *Sagging skin in the temple and surrounding area*

- *Poor posture, which can contribute to the appearance of fine lines and wrinkles*

It is a simple yet effective Face Yoga pose that can help to relieve tension and improve blood circulation in the temple area.

The Temple Toner exercise in Face Yoga primarily targets **the temporalis muscle**, which is a large muscle that covers the sides of the skull above the ears.

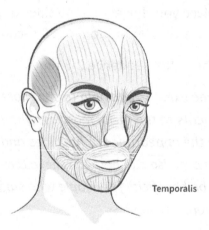

Temporalis

The temporalis muscle is responsible for closing the jaw and moving the lower jaw from side to side. It also plays a role in facial expression and is involved in chewing.

During The Temple Toner exercise, the gentle circular motion applied to the temples and sides of the forehead helps to improve blood flow to the temporalis muscle. This increased blood flow can help to relieve tension and promote relaxation in the muscle, reducing the appearance of fine lines and wrinkles and improving overall facial tone.

It is a non-invasive way to improve the appearance of the cheeks and surrounding area and overall facial appearance.

This is a simple yet effective Face Yoga pose that can help to tone and firm the muscles in the cheeks.

The Cheek Plumper exercise in Face Yoga primarily targets **the buccinator muscle**, which is a flat, thin muscle that runs between the upper and lower jaws, and plays a key role in chewing and facial expression.

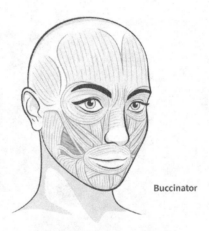

Buccinator

During The Cheek Plumper exercise, the puffing out and moving of air inside the cheeks provides resistance to the buccinator muscle, helping to tone and firm the muscles in the cheeks. This can help to reduce sagging and promote a more youthful appearance in the cheek area.

Additionally, The Cheek Plumper exercise can help to stimulate the flow of oxygen and nutrients to the facial muscles, which can improve skin tone and reduce the appearance of fine lines and wrinkles.

By performing The Cheek Plumper exercise regularly, you can help to maintain healthy facial muscles and reduce the signs of aging in the cheeks. This exercise can also be beneficial for improving the overall health and appearance of the skin in the cheek area.

Here's how to do it:

Apply some facial oil to the palms of your hands and then massage it onto your face and neck, making sure to cover all areas where you will be performing Face Yoga exercises.

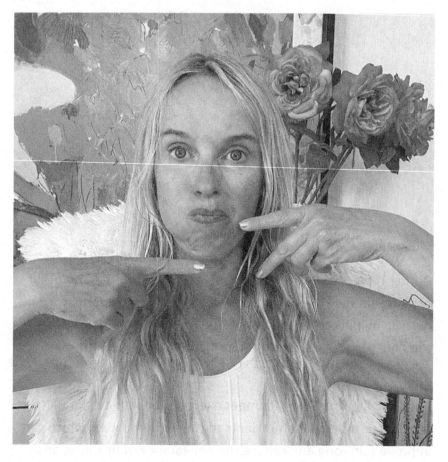

1. Sit in a comfortable position with your back straight and your shoulders relaxed.

2. Take a deep breath and puff out your cheeks.

3. Move the air inside your mouth from one cheek to the other, as if you are swishing mouthwash around in your mouth.

4. Continue moving the air from one cheek to the other for 30 seconds.

5. Relax your cheeks and repeat the exercise 2-3 times.

The Cheek Plumper exercise can help to stimulate the flow of oxygen and nutrients to the facial muscles, which can improve skin tone and reduce the appearance of fine lines and wrinkles. Additionally, this exercise can help to tone and firm the muscles in the cheeks, which can help to reduce sagging and promote a more youthful appearance. By performing The Cheek Plumper exercise regularly, you can help to maintain healthy facial muscles and reduce the signs of aging in the cheeks.

The Neck Smoother

The Neck Smoother is a facial exercise that is designed to help improve the appearance of the neck and surrounding area. It works by exercising the muscles of the neck and surrounding area, which can help to tighten and tone the skin in this area. This exercise can be used to address a variety of face appearance issues, including:

- *Sagging skin in the neck and surrounding area*

- *Poor posture, which can contribute to the appearance of sagging skin*

- *A double chin or excess fat in the neck area*

This is a simple yet effective Face Yoga pose that can help to tone and firm the muscles in the neck and chin.

The Neck Smoother exercise in Face Yoga targets several muscles in the neck and chin area, including the platysma muscle, the sternocleidomastoid muscle, and the digastric muscle.

1. **The platysma muscle** is a thin, flat muscle that runs from the chin to the chest and is responsible for pulling down the corners of the mouth and the skin on the neck.
2. **The sternocleidomastoid muscle** is a long, thin muscle that runs from the base of the skull to the collarbone and is responsible for turning the head and flexing the neck.
3. **The digastric muscle** is a paired muscle located on the underside of the jaw and is responsible for opening the mouth and pulling the jaw downward.

During The Neck Smoother exercise, the chewing motion helps to tone and firm the platysma muscle and the other muscles in the neck and chin area. Additionally, the stretching and turning motions help to improve blood flow to the muscles, which can improve skin tone and reduce the appearance of fine lines and wrinkles.

By performing The Neck Smoother exercise regularly, you can help to maintain healthy facial muscles and reduce the signs of aging in the neck and chin area. This exercise can also be beneficial for improving the overall health and appearance of the skin in the neck and chin area.

Here's how to do it:

Apply some facial oil to the palms of your hands and then massage it onto your face and neck, making sure to cover all

areas where you will be performing Face Yoga exercises.

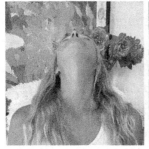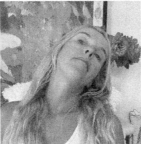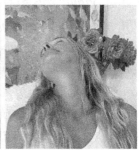

1. Sit in a comfortable position with your back straight and your shoulders relaxed.

2. Tilt your head back and look up at the ceiling.

3. Keeping your lips closed, open your mouth slightly and make a chewing motion with your jaw.

4. Do 20-30 chewing motions, then relax your jaw and return your head to the starting position.

5. Next, tilt your head to the left and try to touch your left ear to your left shoulder.

6. Hold this position for 10-15 seconds, then relax and return your head to the starting position.

7. Repeat on the right side.

8. Finally, turn your head to the left and try to look over your left shoulder.

9. Hold this position for 10-15 seconds, then relax and return your head to the starting position.

10. Repeat on the right side.

The Neck Smoother exercise can help to stimulate the flow of oxygen and nutrients to the facial muscles, which can improve skin tone and reduce the appearance of fine lines and wrinkles. Additionally, this exercise can help to tone and firm the muscles in the neck and chin, which can help to reduce sagging and promote a more youthful appearance. By performing The Neck Smoother exercise regularly, you can help to maintain healthy facial muscles and reduce the signs of aging in the neck and chin area. This exercise can also be beneficial for improving the overall health and appearance of the skin in the neck and chin area.

The Eyebrow Shaper

The Eyebrow Shaper is a facial exercise that is designed to help improve the appearance of the eyebrows and surrounding area. It works by exercising the muscles of the eyebrows and surrounding area, which can help to tighten and tone the skin in this area. This exercise can be used to address a variety of face appearance issues, including:

- *Fine lines and wrinkles in the eyebrow and surrounding area*

- *Sagging skin in the eyebrow and surrounding area*

- *Poor posture, which can contribute to the appearance of fine lines and wrinkles*

This is a simple yet effective Face Yoga pose that can help to tone and lift the muscles around the eyebrows.

The Eyebrow Shaper exercise in Face Yoga primarily targets the frontalis muscle, which is a thin, flat muscle that covers the forehead and extends down to the eyebrows.

The frontalis muscle is responsible for raising the eyebrows and creating horizontal wrinkles on the forehead, commonly known as "worry lines" or "surprise lines."

During The Eyebrow Shaper exercise, the lifting and pressing motion applied to the skin around the eyebrows helps to improve blood flow to **the frontalis muscle**. This increased blood flow can help to tone and lift the muscles around the eyebrows, reducing sagging and promoting a more youthful appearance.

Additionally, The Eyebrow Shaper exercise can help to stimulate the flow of oxygen and nutrients to the facial muscles, which can improve skin tone and reduce the appearance of fine lines and wrinkles.

Here's how to do it:

Apply some facial oil to the palms of your hands and then massage it onto your face and neck, making sure to cover all areas where you will be performing Face Yoga exercises.

1. Sit in a comfortable position with your back straight and your shoulders relaxed.

2. Place your fingertips on the outer edge of your eyebrows.

3. Gently lift your eyebrows upward using your fingertips and hold for 10-15 seconds.

4. Relax your eyebrows and repeat the lifting motion 2-3 times.

5. Next, place your fingertips just above the middle of your eyebrows.

6. Gently press down with your fingertips and try to push your eyebrows downward.

7. Hold this position for 10-15 seconds, then relax and repeat the pressing motion 2-3 times.

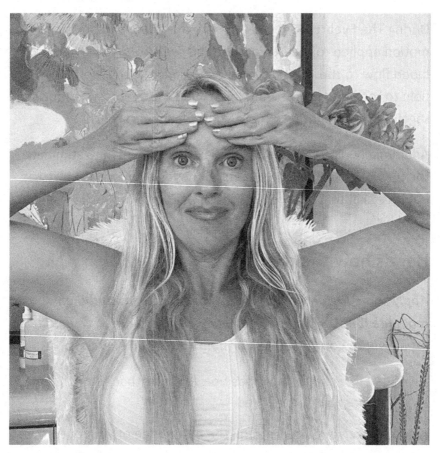

The Eyebrow Shaper exercise can help to stimulate the flow of oxygen and nutrients to the facial muscles, which can improve skin tone and reduce the appearance of fine lines and wrinkles. Additionally, this exercise can help to tone and lift the muscles around the eyebrows, which can help to reduce sagging and promote a more youthful appearance. By performing The Eyebrow Shaper exercise regularly, you can help to maintain healthy facial muscles and reduce the signs of aging around the eyebrows. This exercise can also be beneficial for improving the overall health and

appearance of the skin in the eyebrow area.

The Chin Lift

The Chin Lift is a facial exercise that is designed to help improve the appearance of the chin and surrounding area. It works by exercising the muscles of the chin and surrounding area, which can help to tighten and tone the skin in this area. This exercise can be used to address a variety of face appearance issues, including:

- *Sagging skin in the chin and surrounding area*

- *Poor posture, which can contribute to the appearance of sagging skin*

- *A double chin or excess fat in the chin area*

This simple yet effective Face Yoga pose that can help to tone and firm the muscles in the neck and chin area.

The Chin Lift exercise in Face Yoga targets several muscles in the neck and chin area, including the platysma muscle, the sternocleidomastoid muscle, and the hyoid muscles.

1. **The platysma muscle is** a thin, flat muscle that runs from the chin to the chest and is responsible for pulling down the corners of the mouth and the skin on the neck.
2. **The sternocleidomastoid muscle is** a long, thin muscle that runs from the base of the skull to the collarbone and is responsible for turning the head and flexing the neck.
3. **The hyoid muscles** are a group of small muscles that are located in the neck and are responsible for supporting the hyoid bone, which is an important structure that anchors the tongue and provides support to the muscles in the neck and throat.

During The Chin Lift exercise, the lifting motion helps to tone and firm the platysma muscle and the other muscles in the neck and chin area. Additionally, the stretching and strengthening motions help to improve blood flow to the muscles, which can improve skin tone and reduce the appearance of fine lines and wrinkles.

By performing The Chin Lift exercise regularly, you can help to maintain healthy facial muscles and reduce the signs of aging in the neck and chin area. This exercise can also be beneficial for improving the overall health and appearance of the skin in the neck and chin area.

Here's how to do it:

Apply some facial oil to the palms of your hands and then massage it onto your face and neck, making sure to cover all areas where you will be performing Face Yoga exercises.

1. Sit in a comfortable position with your back straight and your shoulders relaxed.

2. Tilt your head back and look up at the ceiling.

3. Pucker your lips as if you are kissing the ceiling.

4. Hold this position for 5-10 seconds, then relax and return your head to the starting position.

5. Repeat The Chin Lift exercise 5-10 times.

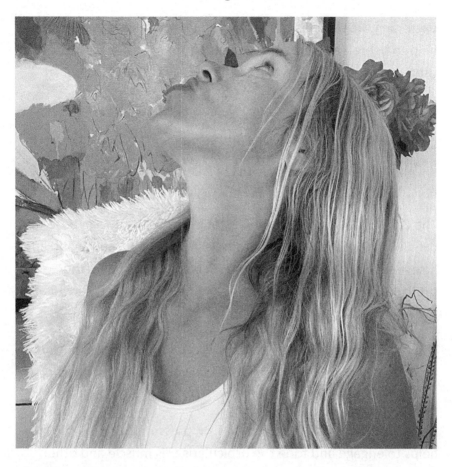

The Chin Lift exercise can help to stimulate the flow of oxygen and nutrients to the facial muscles, which can improve skin tone and reduce the appearance of fine lines and wrinkles. Additionally, this exercise can help to tone and firm the muscles in the neck and chin area, which can help to reduce sagging and promote a more youthful appearance.

The Lip Press

The Lip Press is a facial exercise that is designed to help improve the appearance of the lips and surrounding area. It works by exercising the muscles of the lips and surrounding area, which can help to tighten and tone the skin in this area. This exercise can be used to address a variety of face appearance issues, including:

- *Fine lines and wrinkles in the lips and surrounding area*

- *Sagging skin in the lips and surrounding area*

- *Poor posture, which can contribute to the appearance of fine lines and wrinkles*

The Lip Press exercise is a simple yet effective Face Yoga pose that can help to tone and firm the muscles around the mouth and lips. It several muscles around the mouth and lips, including **the orbicularis oris muscle**, which is a circular muscle that surrounds the mouth.

The orbicularis oris muscle is responsible for closing and puckering the lips, as well as helping to form facial expressions such as smiling and frowning.

During The Lip Press exercise, the firm pressure between the lips helps to engage and tone the orbicularis oris muscle and other muscles around the mouth and lips. Additionally, the stimulation of blood flow to the area can help to improve skin tone and reduce the appearance of fine lines and wrinkles.

Here's how to do it:

Apply some facial oil to the palms of your hands and then massage it onto your face and neck, making sure to cover all areas where you will be performing Face Yoga exercises.

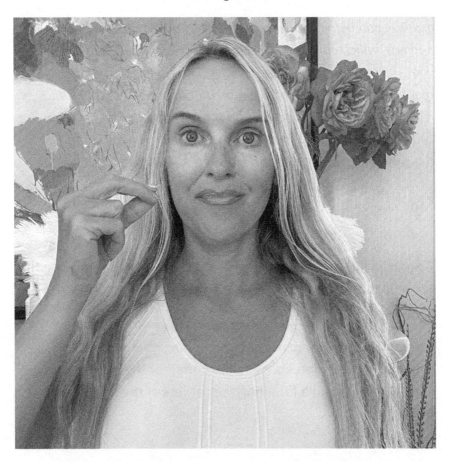

1. Sit in a comfortable position with your back straight and your shoulders relaxed.

2. Close your mouth and press your lips together firmly.

3. Use your facial muscles to smile slightly, while maintaining the firm pressure between your lips.

4. Hold this position for 5-10 seconds, then relax and repeat the exercise 5-10 times.

The Lip Press exercise can help to stimulate the flow of oxygen and nutrients to the facial muscles, which can improve skin tone and reduce the appearance of fine lines and wrinkles. Additionally, this exercise can help to tone and firm the muscles around the mouth and lips, which can help to reduce sagging and promote a more youthful appearance. By performing The Lip Press exercise regularly, you can help to maintain healthy facial muscles and reduce the signs of aging around the mouth and lips. This exercise can also be beneficial for improving the overall health and appearance of the skin in the mouth and lip area.

The Lip Smile

The Lip Smile exercise is a simple yet effective Face Yoga pose that can help to tone and lift the muscles around the mouth and lips.

The Lip Smile exercise in Face Yoga primarily targets **the zygomaticus major muscle**, which is a long, thin muscle that extends from the cheekbone to the corner of the mouth. This muscle is responsible for lifting the corners of the mouth and creating a smile.

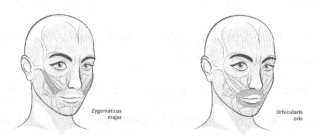

1. **The zygomaticus major muscle** is a long, thin muscle that extends from the cheekbone to the corner of the mouth. This muscle is responsible for lifting the corners of the mouth and creating a smile.
2. **The orbicularis oris muscle** is a circular muscle that surrounds the mouth and is responsible for closing and

puckering the lips, as well as helping to form facial expressions such as smiling and frowning.

Additionally, **the orbicularis oris muscle**, a circular muscle that surrounds the mouth, is also engaged during the The Lip Smile exercise. This muscle is responsible for closing and puckering the lips, as well as helping to form facial expressions such as smiling and frowning.

During The Lip Smile exercise, the stretching and lifting motion helps to tone and lift the zygomaticus major muscle and other muscles around the mouth and lips. Additionally, the stimulation of blood flow to the area can help to improve skin tone and reduce the appearance of fine lines and wrinkles.

Here's how to do it:

Apply some facial oil to the palms of your hands and then massage it onto your face and neck, making sure to cover all areas where you will be performing Face Yoga exercises.

1. Sit in a comfortable position with your back straight and your shoulders relaxed.

2. Place your fingertips at the corners of your mouth.

3. Use your facial muscles to smile as widely as possible, while using your fingertips to lift the corners of your mouth even higher.

4. Hold this position for 5-10 seconds, then relax and repeat the exercise 5-10 times.

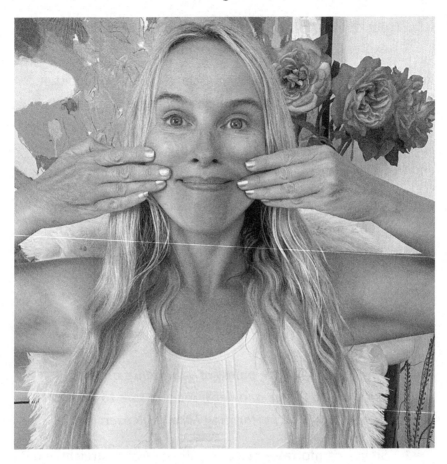

The Lip Smile exercise can help to stimulate the flow of oxygen and nutrients to the facial muscles, which can improve skin tone and reduce the appearance of fine lines and wrinkles. Additionally, this exercise can help to tone and lift the muscles around the mouth and lips, which can help to reduce sagging and promote a more youthful appearance. By performing The Lip Smile exercise regularly, you can help to maintain healthy facial muscles and reduce the signs of aging around the mouth and lips. This exercise can also be beneficial for improving the overall health and appearance of the skin in the mouth and lip area.

The Neck Lift

The Neck Lift is a facial exercise that is designed to help improve the appearance of the neck and surrounding area. It works by exercising the muscles of the neck and surrounding area, which can help to tighten and tone the skin in this area. This exercise can be used to address a variety of face appearance issues, including:

- *Sagging skin in the neck and surrounding area*

- *Poor posture, which can contribute to the appearance of sagging skin*

- *A double chin or excess fat in the neck area*

This is a simple yet effective Face Yoga pose that can help to tone and strengthen the muscles in the neck and jawline.

The Neck Lift exercise in Face Yoga targets several muscles in the neck and jawline area, including the platysma muscle, the sternocleidomastoid muscle, and the hyoid muscles.

1. **The platysma muscle** is a thin, flat muscle that runs from the chin to the chest and is responsible for pulling down the corners of the mouth and the skin on the neck.
2. **The sternocleidomastoid muscle is** a long, thin muscle that runs from the base of the skull to the collarbone and is responsible for turning the head and flexing the neck.
3. **The hyoid muscles** are a group of small muscles that are located in the neck and are responsible for supporting the hyoid bone, which is an important structure that anchors the tongue and provides support to the muscles in the neck and throat.

During The Neck Lift exercise, the pressing of the tongue against the roof of the mouth and the lowering of the chin engages and tones the platysma muscle and the other muscles in the neck and jawline area. Additionally, the stretching and strengthening motions help to improve blood flow to the muscles, which can improve skin tone and reduce the appearance of fine lines and wrinkles.

Here's how to do it:

Apply some facial oil to the palms of your hands and then massage it onto your face and neck, making sure to cover all areas where you will be performing Face Yoga exercises.

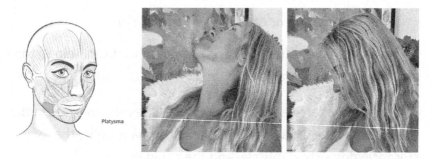

Platysma

1. Sit in a comfortable position with your back straight and your shoulders relaxed.

2. Tilt your head back so that you are looking at the ceiling.

3. Press your tongue to the roof of your mouth and hold it there.

4. Lower your chin toward your chest as far as you can, while keeping your tongue pressed to the roof of your mouth.

5. Hold this position for 5-10 seconds, then relax and return your head to the starting position.

6. Repeat The Neck Lift exercise 5-10 times.

The Neck Lift exercise can help to stimulate the flow of oxygen and nutrients to the facial muscles, which can improve skin tone and reduce the appearance of fine lines and wrinkles. Additionally, this exercise can help to tone and strengthen the muscles in the neck and jawline, which can help to reduce sagging and promote a more youthful appearance. By performing The Neck Lift exercise regularly, you can help to maintain healthy facial muscles and reduce the signs of aging in the neck and jawline. This exercise can also be beneficial for improving the overall health and appearance of the skin in the neck and jawline area.

The Cheekbone Lift

The Cheekbone Lift is a facial exercise that is designed to help improve the appearance of the cheekbones and surrounding area. It works by exercising the muscles of the cheekbones and surrounding area, which can help to tighten and tone the skin in this area. This exercise can be used to address a variety of face appearance issues, including:

- *Sagging skin in the cheekbones and surrounding area*

- *Poor posture, which can contribute to the appearance of sagging skin*

- *Flat or sunken cheekbones, which can contribute to an aged or tired appearance*

This is a simple, yet effective Face Yoga pose that can help to tone and lift the muscles around the cheekbones and eyes.

The Cheekbone Lift exercise in Face Yoga primarily targets the zygomaticus major muscle and the orbicularis oculi muscle.

1. **The zygomaticus major muscle** is a long, thin muscle that extends from the cheekbone to the corner of the mouth. This muscle is responsible for lifting the corners of the mouth and creating a smile, and also helps to lift the skin around the cheekbones when engaged.

2. **The orbicularis oculi muscle** is a circular muscle that surrounds the eye and is responsible for closing and squinting the eye, as well as helping to form facial expressions such as smiling and frowning.

During The Cheekbone Lift exercise, the lifting motion helps to engage and tone the zygomaticus major muscle and other muscles around the cheekbones and eyes, such as the orbicularis oculi muscle. Additionally, the stimulation of blood flow to the area can help to improve skin tone and reduce the appearance of fine lines and wrinkles.

Here's how to do it:

Apply some facial oil to the palms of your hands and then massage it onto your face and neck, making sure to cover all areas where you will be performing Face Yoga exercises.

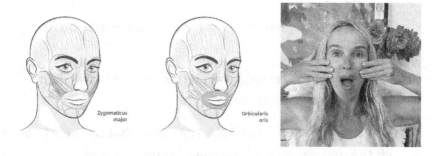

1. Sit in a comfortable position with your back straight and your shoulders relaxed.

2. Use your fingertips to gently lift the skin on your cheekbones upward and outward.

3. Open your mouth and form an "O" shape with your lips.

4. Hold this position for 5-10 seconds, then relax and repeat the exercise 5-10 times.

The Cheekbone Lift exercise can help to stimulate the flow of oxygen and nutrients to the facial muscles, which can improve skin tone and reduce the appearance of fine lines and wrinkles. Additionally, this exercise can help to tone and lift the muscles around the cheekbones and eyes, which can help to reduce sagging and promote a more youthful appearance. By performing The Cheekbone Lift exercise regularly, you can help to maintain healthy facial muscles and reduce the signs of aging around the cheekbones and eyes. This exercise can also be beneficial for improving the overall health and appearance of the skin in the cheek and eye area.

The Mouth Release

The Mouth Release is a facial exercise that is designed to help improve the appearance of the mouth and surrounding area. It works by relaxing the muscles of the mouth and surrounding area, which can help to reduce the appearance of fine lines and wrinkles and improve the overall facial appearance. This exercise can be used to address a variety of face appearance issues, including:

- *Fine lines and wrinkles around the mouth*

- *Tension or tightness in the muscles around the mouth*

- *Poor posture, which can contribute to the appearance of fine lines and wrinkles*

The Mouth Release Facial Yoga Pose is a non-invasive way to improve the appearance of the mouth and surrounding area and overall facial appearance.

It is a simple yet effective Face Yoga pose that can help to relax and relieve tension in the facial muscles around the mouth and jaw.

The Mouth Release exercise in Face Yoga primarily targets the muscles around the mouth and jaw, including the masseter muscle and the orbicularis oris muscle.

1. **The masseter muscle** is a strong muscle that runs along the side of the jaw and is responsible for closing the jaw and clenching the teeth.
2. **The orbicularis oris** muscle is a circular muscle that surrounds the mouth and is responsible for closing and puckering the lips, as well as helping to form facial expressions such as smiling and frowning.

During The Mouth Release exercise, the wide opening of the mouth and the relaxation of the jaw and tongue can help to release tension and stiffness in the masseter muscle and the other muscles around the mouth and jaw.

Additionally, the stimulation of blood flow to the area can help to improve skin tone and reduce the appearance of fine lines and wrinkles.

Here's how to do it:

Apply some facial oil to the palms of your hands and then

massage it onto your face and neck, making sure to cover all areas where you will be performing Face Yoga exercises.

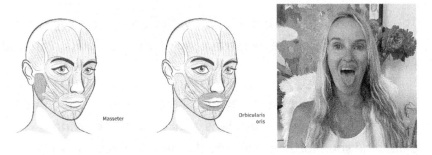

1. Sit in a comfortable position with your back straight and your shoulders relaxed.

2. Open your mouth wide and stick out your tongue as far as you can.

3. Relax your jaw and let it hang loose.

4. Hold this position for 5-10 seconds, then relax and repeat the exercise 5-10 times.

The Mouth Release exercise can help to stimulate the flow of oxygen and nutrients to the facial muscles, which can improve skin tone and reduce the appearance of fine lines and wrinkles. Additionally, this exercise can help to relieve tension and stiffness in the muscles around the mouth and jaw, which can promote a more relaxed and youthful appearance.

By performing The Mouth Release exercise regularly, you can help to maintain healthy facial muscles and reduce the signs of aging around the mouth and jaw. This exercise can also be beneficial for improving the overall health and appearance of the skin in the mouth and jaw area.

The Eye Stretch

The Eye Stretch exercise is a simple yet effective Face Yoga pose that can help to reduce eye strain and improve circulation around the eyes.

The Eye Stretch exercise in Face Yoga targets the muscles around the eyes, including the orbicularis oculi muscle, the levator palpebrae superioris muscle, and the superior rectus muscle.

1. **The orbicularis** oculi muscle is a circular muscle that surrounds the eye and is responsible for closing and squinting the eye, as well as helping to form facial expressions such as smiling and frowning.
2. **The levator palpebrae superioris muscle** is a thin muscle that runs along the upper eyelid and is responsible for lifting the eyelid.
3. **The superior rectus muscle** is a small muscle located in the upper portion of the eye socket and is responsible for elevating the eye and rotating it inward.

During The Eye Stretch exercise, the upward and downward movement of the eyes can help to engage and stretch the orbicularis oculi muscle, while the side-to-side movement can engage and stretch the superior rectus muscle. Additionally, the pressure from the fists against the temples can help to engage the levator palpebrae superioris muscle and promote circulation around the eyes.

By performing The Eye Stretch exercise regularly, you can help to maintain healthy facial muscles and reduce the signs of aging around the eyes. This exercise can also be beneficial for improving the overall health and appearance of the skin in the eye area and reducing eye strain and fatigue.

Here are the steps to perform this exercise:

Apply some facial oil to the palms of your hands and then massage it onto your face and neck, making sure to cover all areas where you will be performing Face Yoga exercises.

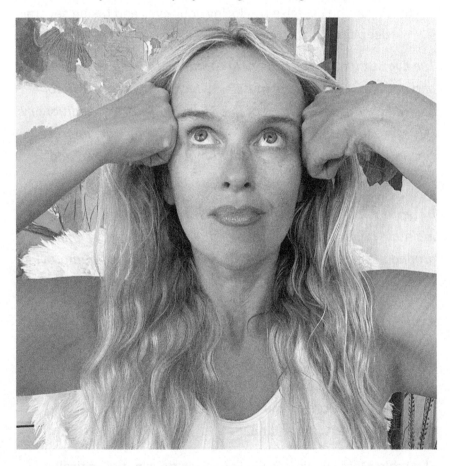

1. Sit in a comfortable position with your back straight and your shoulders relaxed.

2. Make a fist with both hands and place them against your temples.

3. Look straight ahead and focus on a point in front of you.

4. Without moving your head, slowly move your eyes upward as far as you can, then downward as far as you can.

5. Repeat this movement 5-10 times, then relax and repeat the exercise with your eyes moving from side to side.

6. Finish the exercise by closing your eyes and taking several deep breaths.

The Eye Stretch exercise can help to stimulate the flow of oxygen and nutrients to the facial muscles, which can improve skin tone and reduce the appearance of fine lines and wrinkles. Additionally, this exercise can help to reduce eye strain and fatigue, improve circulation around the eyes, and promote a more relaxed and youthful appearance.

By performing The Eye Stretch exercise regularly, you can help to maintain healthy facial muscles and reduce the signs of aging around the eyes. This exercise can also be beneficial for improving the overall health and appearance of the skin in the eye area.

The Scalp Massage

The Scalp Massage exercise is a simple, yet effective Face Yoga pose that can help to stimulate blood flow and promote relaxation in the scalp and head.

The Scalp Massage exercise in Face Yoga does not specifically target any facial muscles. However, it can indirectly benefit the muscles of the face by increasing blood flow and promoting relaxation throughout the scalp and head.

The muscles of the face are supplied by a network of blood

vessels that deliver oxygen and nutrients to the muscles. By increasing blood flow to the scalp through The Scalp Massage exercise, more oxygen and nutrients can be delivered to the facial muscles, which can improve their health and function.

Additionally, tension and stress in the scalp and head can lead to tension in the facial muscles, which can contribute to the formation of fine lines and wrinkles. By promoting relaxation and reducing stress and tension in the scalp and head through The Scalp Massage exercise, the facial muscles can also benefit.

Overall, The Scalp Massage exercise can be a beneficial addition to a Face Yoga routine for promoting overall facial health and relaxation.

Here are the steps to perform this exercise:

Apply some facial oil to the palms of your hands and then massage it onto your scalp, making sure to cover all areas where you will be performing Face Yoga exercises.

1. Sit in a comfortable position with your back straight and your shoulders relaxed.

2. Place your fingertips on your scalp and begin to gently massage your scalp in circular motions.

3. Move your fingertips from the front of your head to the back, covering the entire scalp.

4. Use enough pressure to feel a gentle stretch in the scalp, but not so much that it causes pain.

5. Continue the massage for 1-2 minutes, then relax and take several deep breaths.

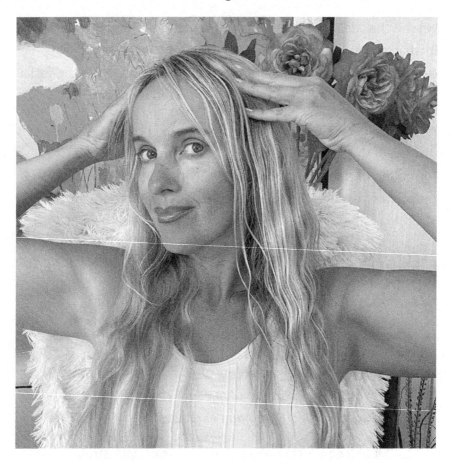

The Scalp Massage exercise can help to stimulate the flow of oxygen and nutrients to the scalp and hair follicles, which can improve the health and appearance of the hair. Additionally, this exercise can help to promote relaxation and reduce stress and tension in the scalp and head.

The Nostril Flare

The Nostril Flare exercise is a simple, yet effective Face Yoga pose that can help to tone and strengthen the muscles around the nostrils and upper lip.

The Nostril Flare exercise in Face Yoga targets the muscles around the nostrils and upper lip, including the nasalis muscle and the levator labii superioris muscle.

The nasalis muscle is a paired muscle located on either side of the nose and is responsible for flaring the nostrils.

The levator labii superioris muscle is a thin muscle that runs from the upper lip to the base of the nose and is responsible for lifting the upper lip and creating facial expressions such as a smile or a snarl.

During The Nostril Flare exercise, the flaring of the nostrils engages and tones the nasalis muscle, while the inhalation and holding of the breath can engage and tone the levator labii superioris muscle. Additionally, the stimulation of blood flow to the area can help to improve skin tone and reduce the appearance of fine lines and wrinkles.

Here are the steps to perform this exercise:

Apply some facial oil to the palms of your hands and then massage it onto your face and neck, making sure to cover all areas where you will be performing Face Yoga exercises.

1. Sit in a comfortable position with your back straight and your shoulders relaxed.

2. Place your fingertips on your cheeks, just below the eyes.

3. Inhale deeply through your nose, then flare your nostrils and hold the breath for a few seconds.

4. Exhale through your mouth, making a "ha" sound.

5. Repeat this exercise 5-10 times.

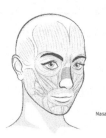 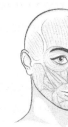 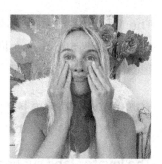

Nasalis

Levator
labii superioris
alaeque nasi

The Nostril Flare exercise can help to stimulate the flow of oxygen and nutrients to the facial muscles, which can improve skin tone and reduce the appearance of fine lines and wrinkles. Additionally, this exercise can help to tone and strengthen the muscles around the nostrils and upper lip, which can help to reduce sagging and promote a more youthful appearance.

By performing The Nostril Flare exercise regularly, you can help to maintain healthy facial muscles and reduce the signs of aging around the nostrils and upper lip. This exercise can also be beneficial for improving the overall health and appearance of the skin in the nose and upper lip area.

The Eyelid Strengthen

The Eyelid Strengthen exercise is a simple yet effective Face Yoga pose that can help to strengthen the muscles around the eyes and improve the appearance of the eyelids.

The Eyelid Strengthen exercise in Face Yoga targets the muscles around the eyes, including the orbicularis oculi muscle, the levator palpebrae superioris muscle, and the superior tarsal muscle.

1. **The orbicularis oculi muscle** is a circular muscle that surrounds the eye and is responsible for closing and

squinting the eye, as well as helping to form facial expressions such as smiling and frowning.

2. **The levator palpebrae superioris muscle is** a thin muscle that runs along the upper eyelid and is responsible for lifting the eyelid.

3. **The superior tarsal muscle** is a small muscle located in the upper eyelid and is responsible for helping to open the eyelid.

During The Eyelid Strengthen exercise, the gentle pressure of the fingers on the eyelids can help to engage and tone the orbicularis oculi muscle, while the lifting and lowering of the eyelids can engage and tone the levator palpebrae superioris muscle and the superior tarsal muscle. Additionally, the stimulation of blood flow to the area can help to improve skin tone and reduce the appearance of fine lines and wrinkles.

Here are the steps to perform this exercise:

Apply some facial oil to the palms of your hands and then massage it onto your face and neck, making sure to cover all areas where you will be performing Face Yoga exercises.

1. Sit in a comfortable position with your back straight and your shoulders relaxed.

2. Close your eyes and place your index fingers on your eyelids.

3. Gently press your eyelids down against your fingers, then release.

4. Repeat this exercise 10-20 times.

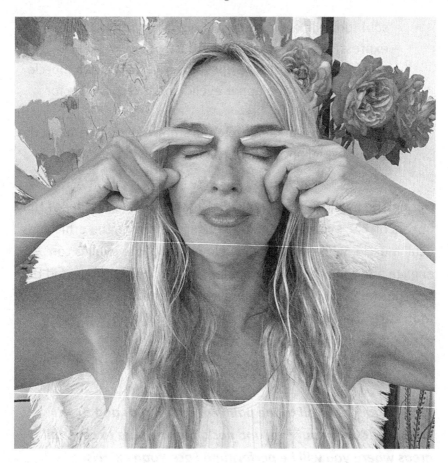

The Eyelid Strengthen exercise can help to stimulate the flow of oxygen and nutrients to the facial muscles, which can improve skin tone and reduce the appearance of fine lines and wrinkles. Additionally, this exercise can help to strengthen the muscles around the eyes, which can help to reduce sagging and promote a more youthful appearance.

By performing The Eyelid Strengthen exercise regularly, you can help to maintain healthy facial muscles and reduce the signs of aging around the eyes. This exercise can also be beneficial for improving the overall health and appearance of the skin in the eye area.

The Tongue Scrub

The Tongue Scrub exercise is a simple, yet effective Face Yoga pose that can help to improve oral hygiene, freshen breath, and tone the muscles around the mouth and tongue.

The Tongue Scrub exercise in Face Yoga does not specifically target any facial muscles. However, it can indirectly benefit the muscles of the face by promoting oral hygiene and improving the health and appearance of the tongue and mouth.

The muscles of the face are supplied by a network of blood vessels that deliver oxygen and nutrients to the muscles. By promoting oral hygiene and removing bacteria and debris from the tongue through The Tongue Scrub exercise, more oxygen and nutrients can be delivered to the facial muscles, which can improve their health and function.

Additionally, tension and stress in the tongue and mouth can lead to tension in the facial muscles, which can contribute to the formation of fine lines and wrinkles. By promoting relaxation and reducing stress and tension in the tongue and mouth area through The Tongue Scrub exercise, the facial muscles can also benefit.

Overall, The Tongue Scrub exercise can be a beneficial addition to a Face Yoga routine for promoting overall facial health and oral hygiene.

Here are the steps to perform this exercise:

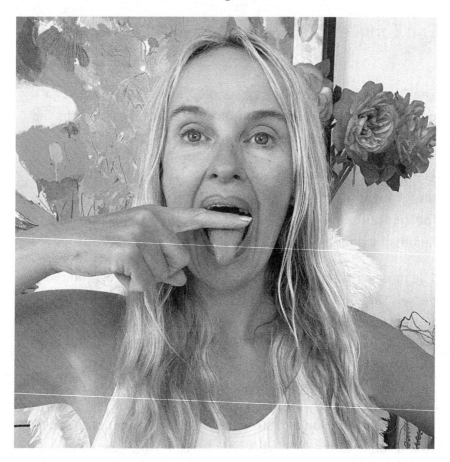

1. Sit in a comfortable position with your back straight and your shoulders relaxed.

2. Stick out your tongue as far as you can.

3. Use your fingers or a tongue scraper to gently scrub your tongue from the back to the front.

4. Repeat this scrubbing motion 5-10 times.

5. Finish the exercise by rinsing your mouth with water.

The Tongue Scrub exercise can help to remove bacteria and debris from the tongue, which can improve oral hygiene and freshen breath.

Additionally, this exercise can help to tone the muscles around the mouth and tongue, which can help to reduce sagging and promote a more youthful appearance. By performing The Tongue Scrub exercise regularly, you can help to maintain healthy facial muscles and reduce the signs of aging around the mouth and tongue area. This exercise can also be beneficial for improving oral hygiene and freshening breath.

The Temple Release

The Temple Release exercise is a simple, yet effective Face Yoga pose that can help to relieve tension and reduce stress in the temples and forehead.

It does not specifically target any facial muscles. However, it can indirectly benefit the muscles of the face by promoting relaxation and reducing tension and stress in the temples and forehead.

The muscles of the face are supplied by a network of blood vessels that deliver oxygen and nutrients to the muscles. By promoting relaxation and increasing blood flow to the temples and forehead through The Temple Release exercise, more oxygen and nutrients can be delivered to the facial muscles, which can improve their health and function.

Additionally, tension and stress in the temples and forehead can lead to tension in the facial muscles, which can contribute to the formation of fine lines and wrinkles. By promoting relaxation and reducing stress and tension in the temples and forehead area through The Temple Release exercise, the facial muscles can also benefit.

Overall, The Temple Release exercise can be a beneficial addition to a Face Yoga routine for promoting overall facial health and relaxation. It can also help to reduce stress and tension in the face and scalp and promote a more youthful appearance.

Here are the steps to perform this exercise:

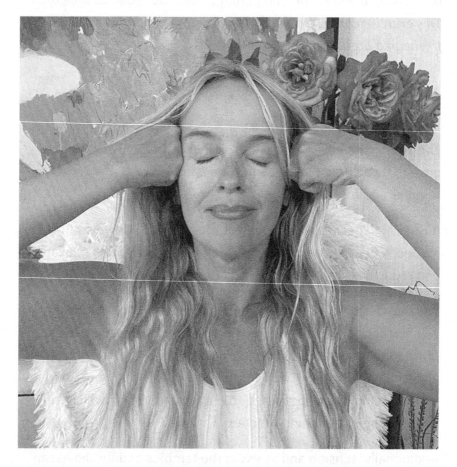

Apply some facial oil to the palms of your hands and then massage it onto your face and neck, making sure to cover all areas where you will be performing Face Yoga exercises.

1. Sit in a comfortable position with your back straight and your shoulders relaxed.

2. Place your fingertips on your temples.

3. Close your eyes and take several deep breaths.

4. Apply gentle pressure to your temples with your fingertips and hold for 10-20 seconds.

5. Release the pressure and take several deep breaths.

6. Repeat this exercise 5-10 times.

The Temple Release exercise can help to stimulate blood flow and promote relaxation in the temples and forehead. Additionally, this exercise can help to reduce tension and stress in the muscles of the face and scalp, which can contribute to the formation of fine lines and wrinkles. By performing The Temple Release exercise regularly, you can help to maintain healthy facial muscles and reduce the signs of aging around the temples and forehead. This exercise can also be beneficial for reducing stress and tension in the face and promoting relaxation.

A Step-by-Step Guide to a Sample Face Yoga Practice

Here is a sample Face Yoga routine that incorporates the use of face oils:

1. **The Brow Smoother:** Apply a drop of your favorite face oil to your fingertips and gently massage into the skin between your eyebrows. Place your fingers on the inner corners of your eyebrows and gently pull the skin towards your temples. While holding the skin taut, raise your eyebrows as high as you can. Hold for a few seconds and then release. Repeat 10 times.
2. **The Cheek Plumper:** Apply a drop of face oil to your fingertips and massage into your cheeks using upward and outward motions. Pucker your lips and suck in your cheeks. Hold this position for 5 seconds and then release. Repeat 10 times.
3. **The Neck Lift:** Apply a drop of face oil to your fingertips and massage into your neck using upward and outward motions. Tilt your head back and look up at the ceiling. Press your tongue to the roof of your mouth and hold for 5 seconds. Release and repeat 10 times.
4. **The Temple Toner:** Apply a drop of face oil to your fingertips and gently massage into your temples. Close your eyes and breathe deeply. Hold for 30 seconds and then release.
5. **The Lip Press:** Apply a drop of face oil to your fingertips and massage into your lips using circular motions. Place your lips together and apply gentle pressure. Hold for 5 seconds and then release. Repeat 10 times.

6. **The Eye Stretch:** Apply a drop of face oil to your fingertips and gently massage into the skin around your eyes. Place your index fingers under your eyebrows and gently lift the skin upwards. While holding the skin taut, look up towards the ceiling. Hold for 5 seconds and then release. Repeat 10 times.

7. **The Chin Lift:** Apply a drop of face oil to your fingertips and massage into your chin and jawline using upward and outward motions. Tilt your head back and press your tongue to the roof of your mouth. Hold for 5 seconds and then release. Repeat 10 times.

8. **The Nostril Flare:** Inhale deeply and apply a drop of face oil to your fingertips. Gently massage into the skin around your nose. Flare your nostrils as wide as you can. Hold for 5 seconds and then release. Repeat 10 times.

9. **The Mouth Release:** Apply a drop of face oil to your fingertips and massage into your cheeks using circular motions. Open your mouth wide and stick out your tongue as far as you can. Hold for 5 seconds and then release. Repeat 10 times.

10. **The Scalp Massage:** Apply a few drops of face oil to your fingertips and gently massage into your scalp in circular motions. Focus on the areas where you hold tension. Continue for 1-2 minutes.

Remember to breathe deeply and slowly throughout the routine, and to practice each pose with gentle and controlled movements. By using face oils in combination with Face Yoga, you can enhance the benefits for your skin, nourishing and hydrating your skin while promoting a more youthful and radiant complexion.

A Step-by-Step Guide to a Morning Face Yoga, Oil, and Massage Routine.

Facial yoga, when combined with facial massage and the use of face oils, can be an effective way to enhance the appearance of your skin and improve its overall health. This routine can be performed in the morning to start your day off feeling refreshed and rejuvenated. Below is a step-by-step guide to a sample Face Yoga practice with a face oil and face massage routine.

Step 1: Cleanse Your Face Begin by thoroughly washing your face with a gentle cleanser to remove any impurities or excess oil. This will help to prepare your skin for the yoga and massage routine.

Step 2: Apply Face Oil Once your face is clean and dry, place a small amount of face oil onto the palms of your hands and gently massage it into your skin. Make sure to cover your entire face and neck, including the areas where you will be performing the yoga exercises.

Step 3: Warm-Up Exercises Start with some simple warm-up exercises to get your facial muscles moving and to increase circulation. Gently massage your forehead, temples, and cheekbones to loosen up your skin and prepare for the yoga exercises.

Step 4: Facial Yoga Exercises Perform a series of facial yoga exercises, focusing on different areas of your face and neck. Some popular facial yoga exercises include:

- **Forehead Smoothing:** Place your index fingers on your temples and gently smooth out any wrinkles on your forehead.

- **Smile and Hold**: Smile as widely as you can and hold for a few seconds.

- **Cheek Lift:** Place your index and middle fingers under your cheekbones and gently lift your cheeks.

- **Neck Stretch:** Tilt your head back and stretch your neck, holding for a few seconds.

Step 5: Face Massage After completing the yoga exercises, it's time to give your skin a little extra love with a facial massage. Use your fingers to gently massage your face, starting from your forehead and working your way down to your neck. Pay special attention to any areas that feel tight or tense.

Step 6: Finish with a Cooling Compress To help reduce puffiness and inflammation, finish your routine by applying a cool compress to your face. Simply wet a washcloth with cold water and place it over your face for a few minutes.

That's it! By incorporating this simple Face Yoga, oil, and massage routine into your morning routine, you can give your skin the care and attention it deserves, leaving you feeling refreshed and rejuvenated for the day ahead. Remember to be gentle with your skin and never pull or tug at it, as this can cause damage.

A Step-by-Step Guide to an Evening Face Yoga, Oil, and Massage Routine.

Facial yoga, combined with the use of face oils and facial massage, can be a great way to unwind and relax after a long day, while also improving the health and appearance of your skin. Below is a step-by-step guide to a sample Face Yoga practice with a face oil and face massage routine to perform in the evening.

Step 1: Remove Makeup and Cleanse Your Face Before starting your routine, remove any makeup and thoroughly wash your face with a gentle cleanser to remove any impurities or excess oil. This will help to prepare your skin for the yoga and massage routine.

Step 2: Apply Face Oil Once your face is clean and dry, place a small amount of face oil onto the palms of your hands and gently massage it into your skin. Make sure to cover your entire face and neck, including the areas where you will be performing the yoga exercises.

Step 3: Warm-Up Exercises Start with some simple warm-up exercises to get your facial muscles moving and to increase circulation. Gently massage your forehead, temples, and cheekbones to loosen up your skin and prepare for the yoga exercises.

Step 4: Facial Yoga Exercises Perform a series of facial yoga exercises, focusing on different areas of your face and neck. Some popular facial yoga exercises include:

- **Lion's Face:** Open your mouth wide and stick out your tongue, inhale deeply, then exhale with a "ha" sound.

- **Forehead Wrinkle Release:** Place your fingers on your temples and use circular motions to smooth out wrinkles on your forehead.
- **Crow's Feet Smoothing:** Place your index fingers at the outer corners of your eyes and use circular motions to smooth out wrinkles.
- **Double Chin Tuck:** Tilt your head back and tuck in your chin, hold for a few seconds, then release.

Step 5: Face Massage After completing the yoga exercises, it's time to give your skin a little extra love with a facial massage. Use your fingers to gently massage your face, starting from your forehead and working your way down to your neck. Pay special attention to any areas that feel tight or tense.

Step 6: Finish with a Relaxing Compress To help you relax and unwind, finish your routine by applying a warm compress to your face. Simply wet a washcloth with warm water and place it over your face for a few minutes.

That's it! By incorporating this simple Face Yoga, oil, and massage routine into your evening routine, you can give your skin the care and attention it deserves, while also helping to relieve stress and promote relaxation. Remember to be gentle with your skin and never pull or tug at it, as this can cause damage.

Conclusion: Unlocking the Benefits of Face Yoga and Face Oils: Achieving a Healthier, More Youthful-looking Complexion with Daily Practice.

In conclusion, Face Yoga and face oils can offer numerous benefits for the skin, including improved circulation, toning of facial muscles, reduced signs of aging, and increased relaxation and stress relief. By incorporating these practices into your daily skincare routine, you can achieve a healthier, more youthful-looking complexion that glows from within.

Remember to choose face oils that are suitable for your skin type and incorporate them into your skincare routine according to your specific needs. Similarly, practice Face Yoga consistently and regularly for maximum benefits.

It's important to note that while Face Yoga and face oils can provide excellent benefits, they are not a replacement for a healthy diet, exercise, and good skincare habits. Eating a balanced diet, getting enough sleep, and protecting your skin from sun damage are also essential for maintaining a healthy complexion.

Incorporating Face Yoga and face oils into your skincare routine can provide a natural and effective way to nourish, hydrate, and protect your skin. By practicing Face Yoga regularly, you can help to tone and strengthen the muscles in your face, reducing the appearance of fine lines and wrinkles and promoting a more youthful and radiant complexion.

When used in conjunction with Face Yoga, face oils can provide additional benefits for your skin. Oils like jojoba oil, rosehip oil, argan oil, marula oil, and plum seed oil can help to nourish and hydrate the skin, improve skin texture and tone, and promote overall facial health. By selecting the right face oil for your skin type and concerns and applying it correctly using gentle massaging and acupressure techniques, you can enhance the benefits of your Face Yoga practice.

Eating a balanced diet, drinking plenty of water, getting enough sleep, and reducing stress can all contribute to overall skin health and wellness. Additionally, it is important to use sun protection when spending time outdoors, as face oils do not provide any protection against UV rays.

In conclusion, incorporating Face Yoga and face oils into your skincare routine can provide a natural and holistic approach to achieving healthy, radiant, and youthful-looking skin. By practicing Face Yoga regularly and using the right face oil for your skin type and concerns, you can nourish, hydrate, and protect your skin from the inside out. When used in combination with a healthy lifestyle and sun protection, Face Yoga and face oils can help you achieve your best skin yet.

ABOUT THE AUTHOR

Maia Sobinina is a certified Zumba instructor and skincare expert with over 10 of experience in the industry.

In addition to her passion for skincare, Maia holds two Master's degrees in Advertising and Energy Finance from the University of Texas at Austin. Her love for education has driven her to dedicate her life to researching natural skincare, healthy living, and happiness. Maia is the founder of the brand "Girls are Gorgeous" which is dedicated to researching and producing chemical-free, plant-powered skincare products. With her extensive knowledge and experience, Maia is a trusted expert in the field of natural skincare and wellness.

With a strive for helping others achieve their best skin, Maia Sobinina has dedicated their career to studying the connection between facial exercises, face oils and skin health. In Maia's Face Yoga Book, they share their expertise and knowledge on the topic, providing a comprehensive guide to facial exercises and the use of face oils for a more youthful, radiant complexion.

Maia has a following of dedicated fans and students who have seen positive results from incorporating their techniques into their skincare routine. Get ready to transform your skin with Maia's expert guidance in "Face Yoga Book."

Keep informed about our newest and updated developments by scanning this QR code.